SUCCESSFUL AGING

SUCCESSFUL AGING

JOHN W. ROWE, M.D.
AND ROBERT L. KAHN, PH.D.

Pantheon Books   *New York*

This book is designed to provide accurate and authoritative information regarding the subject matters covered. It is published with the understanding that in this book the authors are not engaged in rendering medical or other professional services. If an individual is considering changes in his or her health-related practices or regimens, then medical advice or other expert assistance is required, and the services of a competent physician or other professional person should be sought.

Copyright © 1998 by John Wallis Rowe, M.D., and Robert L. Kahn, Ph.D.

All rights reserved under International and Pan-American Copyright Conventions. Published in the United States by Pantheon Books, a division of Random House, Inc., New York, and simultaneously in Canada by Random House of Canada Limited, Toronto.

Library of Congress Cataloging-in-Publication Data

Rowe, John W. (John Wallis), 1944–
Successful aging / John W. Rowe, and Robert L. Kahn.
p.   cm.
Includes bibliographical references and index.
ISBN 0-375-40045-1
1. Longevity.   2. Aging.   I. Kahn, Robert Louis, 1918–   .
II. Title.
QP85.R69   1998
613'.0438—dc21   97-36900
CIP

Random House Web Address: http://www.randomhouse.com

Book design by Trina Stahl

Printed in the United States of America
First Edition
2   4   6   8   9   7   5   3   1

To Beatrice and Valerie

Contents

Contents

ACKNOWLEDGMENTS

Three groups of colleagues have made this book possible. First we are exceptionally grateful to the board and staff of the John D. and Catherine T. MacArthur Foundation, including John Corbally, who served as president of the foundation at the inception of our efforts, and Adele Simmons, his successor, for their unwavering support of our mission to launch a major research program in a new area—Successful Aging. The staff of the foundation's Health Program, including William Bevan, Denis Prager, Robert Rose, Idy Gitelson, Laurie Garduque, and Ruth Runeborg, were extraordinary in their guidance, support, and encouragement over the course of a decade. Our fellow members of the Successful Aging Network, listed individually in the Foreword, are a remarkable interdisciplinary group of distinguished scientists and collaborators. It has been a great privilege for us to work with them—this book is as much theirs as it is ours.

Our special thanks to a trio of exceptionally talented colleagues and mentors who patiently led two scientists through the process of converting a body of research to a volume for a general audience. Amanda Urban's vision, expertise, and enthusiasm sparked this project and made it happen. Linda Healey, our supportive, insightful editor at Pantheon, had a significant impact on the organization and clarity of this book. Our collaborator, Tracy Chutorian Semler, is a truly remarkable colleague whose intelligence, energy, and enthusiasm were critical to this effort.

Lastly, we express our deep appreciation to Dr. Eileen Callahan, who was so very helpful in the literature review, and to Robin Lounsbury, Lisa Gambino, and Maribel Sanchez for their exceptional skill, patience, and good humor through the production of numerous drafts of the manuscript.

We have been tremendously fortunate to work with these outstanding colleagues and are deeply appreciative to each of them for their important contributions.

FOREWORD

TOWARD A NEW GERONTOLOGY
The MacArthur Foundation Study of Successful Aging

This book deals with three fundamental questions about human aging: What does it mean to age successfully? What can each of us do to be successful at this most important life task? What changes in American society will enable more men and women to age successfully?

Throughout the 1970s and early 1980s, interest in gerontology (the study of aging) and geriatrics (health care of older persons) was fueled by recognition of the social, economic, and health care consequences of the unprecedented aging of America's population. Despite this energy, the progress of gerontology began to stall in the mid-1980s. Lacking was the conceptual foundation required to understand aging in all its aspects—biological, psychological, and social. There was a persistent preoccupation with disability, disease, and chronological age, rather than with the positive aspects of aging. This negative perspective was coupled with a serious underestimation of the effects of lifestyle and other psychosocial factors on the well-being of older persons. It was in this context that the MacArthur Study was born.

In 1984, the John D. and Catherine T. MacArthur Foundation assembled a group of scholars from major disciplines relevant to aging to develop the conceptual basis of a "new gerontology." The project: Conduct a long-term research program to gather the knowledge needed to improve older Americans' physical and mental abilities.

Our group consisted of sixteen scientists drawn from biology, neuroscience, neuropsychology, epidemiology, sociology, genetics, psychology, neurology, physiology, and geriatric medicine. We were committed to an interdisciplinary research program, and set out to chart a course to provide fresh insights into aging in America. The members of the MacArthur group, our disciplines, and current academic locations are listed at the end of this foreword.

The MacArthur Study (which was actually a coherent set of dozens of individual research projects) was rooted in our concept of "successful aging"—that is, the many factors which permit individuals to continue to function effectively, both physically and mentally, in old age. We emphasized the *positive aspects of aging*—which had been terribly overlooked. The goal was to move beyond the limited view of chronological age and to clarify the genetic, biomedical, behavioral, and social factors responsible for retaining—and even enhancing—people's ability to function in later life. In sum, we were trying to pinpoint the many factors that conspire to put one octogenarian on cross-country skis and another in a wheelchair. We outline the key elements of successful aging in chapter 2, and elaborate on each throughout the book.

We faced a major hurdle in the historically negative view of aging promoted by both science and society. But we were able to overcome it, in large part, because of the financial commitment on the part of the MacArthur Foundation—which provided well over ten million dollars in support. The research projects took several forms, including studies of over a thousand high-functioning older people for eight years, to determine the factors that predict successful physical and mental aging; detailed studies of hundreds of pairs of Swedish twins to determine the genetic and lifestyle contributions to aging; laboratory-based studies of the responses of older persons to stress; and nearly a dozen studies of brain aging in humans and animals. For ten years, the MacArthur group met at approximately 2- to 3-month intervals to continue ongoing conceptual and method-ological discussions, receive updates on individual research projects, and analyze research data.

When we started the MacArthur Study, interdisciplinary re-search was sorely lacking in the field of gerontology. Experts from different disciplines took part in separate, parallel research efforts, rather than working together to find more meaningful answers. But before long, researchers in all fields were finding that the tools of their own individual trades—from basic biologic research, to the behavioral and social sciences—were inadequate to fully address the critical issues. The MacArthur Foundation sought to establish authentic interdisciplinary science through prolonged, intensive col-laboration. Working in concert, members of the MacArthur group moved beyond defending their own disciplinary bastions and strove instead to reach out and exchange concepts, methods, and tax-onomies. We worked toward a positive understanding of one central theme—effective functioning in later life—from each of our own perspectives.

The speed and effectiveness of the reorientation toward "suc-cessful aging" as a major theme of the "new gerontology" is evident in many ways. The first step—breaking out of the disease frame-work and redefining successful aging—appeared in the journal *Sci-ence* in 1987. Nearly one hundred scientific publications related to the study have followed, and successful aging has since been adopted as a theme of several major national and international meetings, including the Annual Meeting of the Gerontological Society of America, the world's largest group of scholars in gerontology. European research groups, including the Max Planck Institute on Human Development in Berlin and the Nordic Twin Registries, have dedicated their efforts increasingly toward studies of success-ful aging. The World Health Organization Global Program on

Aging has initiated a broad-based study of successful aging in seven countries.

But perhaps the single greatest impact of the MacArthur initiative has been on the National Research Agenda on Aging, recently developed by the Institute of Medicine of the National Academy of Sciences. This blueprint for research in gerontology and geriatrics for the next decade strongly reflects the MacArthur program perspective. The National Institute on Aging and other units of the National Institutes of Health have established funded research programs aimed at understanding successful aging. In 1995 the contributions of the MacArthur Study of aging were recognized with the Allied-Signal Award.

This book brings together our new knowledge about what it takes to age successfully. We place this information from the Mac-Arthur Study in the context of the facts about aging in America. The results of this research provide strategies for middle-aged and older individuals to boost their chance of aging successfully, and it provides the basis for developing effective policies for the successful aging of our society.

THE MacARTHUR FOUNDATION RESEARCH NETWORK ON SUCCESSFUL AGING

John W. Rowe, M.D. (Chair),
geriatrician, physiologist
Mount Sinai Medical Center and
School of Medicine

Marilyn Albert, Ph.D.,
neuropsychologist
Massachusetts General Hospital
Harvard Medical School

Lisa F. Berkman, Ph.D.,
epidemiologist
Harvard School of Public Health

Dan Blazer, M.D., Ph.D.,
geriatric psychiatrist,
epidemiologist
Duke University School of
Medicine

Gilbert Brim, Ph.D.,
social scientist
formerly President of the Russell
Sage Foundation and Foundation
for Child Development

Carl Cotman, Ph.D.,
neurobiologist
University of California, Irvine

David L. Featherman, Ph.D.,
sociologist
Institute for Social Research
University of Michigan

Caleb E. Finch, Ph.D.,
gerontologist, neurobiologist
Andrus Gerontology Center
University of Southern
California

Norman Garmezy, Ph.D.,
psychologist
University of Minnesota

Robert Kahn, Ph.D.,
social psychologist
Institute for Social Research
University of Michigan

Gerald McClearn, Ph.D.,
geneticist
College of Health and Human
Development
Pennsylvania State University

Guy McKhaan, M.D.,
neurologist
The Mind/Brain Institute
Johns Hopkins University

Richard Mohs, Ph.D.,
neuropsychologist
Mount Sinai School of Medicine

John Nesselroade, Ph.D.,
psychologist, statistician
University of Virginia

Edward Schneider, M.D.,
cell biologist, gerontologist,
geneticist
Andrus Gerontology Center
University of Southern California

Teresa Seeman, Ph.D.,
sociologist, epidemiologist
Andrus Gerontology Center
University of Southern California

SUCCESSFUL AGING

AGING IN AMERICA—THE NEW LONGEVITY

THE LEGENDARY BREVITY and astringency of Maine speech has generated a large lexicon of jokes and stories. One of our favorites involves the following two-line exchange between an eager young sociologist and the elderly survey respondent that he is attempting to interview:

> INTERVIEWER: *"Well, old-timer, about what would you say is the death rate around here?"*
> RESPONDENT (after a long pause): *"I'd say about one per person."*

This statistic has not changed. But what has changed and changed dramatically is life expectancy, that is, the expected length of an individual's life from a given point in time. It is estimated that in the forty-five hundred years from the Bronze Age to the year 1900, life expectancy increased twenty-seven years, and that in the short period from 1900 to 1990 it increased by at least that much. The changes have been so dramatic that it is currently estimated that of all the human beings who have ever lived to be sixty-five years or older, half are currently alive.

As we prepare to enter the twenty-first century, previously unimagined numbers of people are growing to be very old in America. Increases in the number and proportion of our population over age sixty-five, and the dynamic changes within the aging population itself, represent perhaps the most dramatic change in American society in this century. And projections call for additional dramatic "graying" of America well into the twenty-first century. At the turn of this century, approximately 4 percent of the United States population was over age sixty-five. Today, that percentage has climbed to 13 percent. More than 70 percent of people now live to the traditional retirement age of sixty-five, nearly three times as many as did so at the turn of the century. Life expectancy at birth in the United States has increased from forty-seven years in 1900 to approximately seventy-six years today. Life expectancy at age sixty-five for the average American is now seventeen years, a full five years longer than at the turn of the century. While the entire population of the United States has tripled since the turn of the century, the absolute number of older persons, currently thirty-three million, has increased elevenfold. The well-known but still unexplained difference in life expectancy of men and women continues, however, with women living about seven years longer than men. There are also striking and disturbing racial differences in life expectancy. Caucasian women, on average, live six years longer than women of African-American descent; Caucasian men live about eight years longer than African-American men.

There have been two major phases in the improvement of life expectancy during the past two centuries. The first was a reduction in infant mortality and death rates in childhood in the nineteenth and early twentieth centuries; the second, a more recent decrease in death rates among middle-aged and older people. Improvements in life expectancy for children are largely due to better prenatal and perinatal care, availability of clean water, increases in food supply, and control of infectious diseases such as smallpox, yellow fever, tuberculosis, and fatal forms of pneumonia. Ninety-eight out of 100 babies born today in the most prosperous nations will live into adulthood. Accidents and, especially in the United States, homicides are now greater dangers to young people than infectious diseases. A direct effect of reduction in childhood death rates is an increase in the proportion of the population that survives to later ages. In the year 1900, only 19 percent of the individuals who died were over age sixty-five. Today, 72 percent of the deaths occur in that age group. Fifty-eight percent of women born in 1900 survived to age sixty-five, and 25 percent survived to age eighty-five. Of women born in the year 1990, almost 90 percent are expected to live to age sixty-five, and more than half will live to age eighty-five.

The second important phase of increasing life expectancy has evolved over the past several decades. It involves a decline in death rates among middle-aged and older individuals. Death rates have declined within the aged population and are now less than half what they were in the year 1900. These advances are related to two key factors: one, people are taking better care of themselves, and two, science and medicine are taking better care of people. For instance, control of chronic or fatal disorders such as hypertension and kidney disease has significantly lowered the risk of death. And the dramatic technological advances in the management of heart disease—the most common killer of men and women in America—have also cut the death rate. Advances in the treatment of heart disease include not only effective medications, but also the development of procedures such as coronary angiography, angioplasty, and new, highly effective approaches to cardiac surgery. Partly as a result of these advances, the old-old—those over age seventy-five—now represent the fastest-growing segment of our population. Finally, alongside the declines in death rates, birth rates have also fallen, as the technological advancement and general prosperity that contribute to longer life have also made contraception widely available.

THE LIMIT OF HUMAN LIFE SPAN

A by-product of this new longevity is a remarkable increase in the number of individuals living to be 100. While centenarians were rare in 1900, their numbers swelled to 32,000 by 1982, 61,000 today, and it is projected that by the middle of the next century, there will be over 600,000 individuals in the United States over the age of 100! Four out of five centenarians are women.

Success in extending life has not reduced the appetite for further gains. It has, however, brought into prominence the question of ultimate limits: Is there some species-determined limit to the number of years human beings can live?

We have only tentative—and controversial—answers to that question. The biblical reference to "three-score and ten" as the appropriate span of human life is often quoted, but the average modern American has already exceeded that limit, and there are biblical examples, from Abraham to Methuselah, of people who attained far greater ages. Some optimistic geriatricians have proposed 120 years as the potential human life span, in the absence of accident or disease. Interestingly, this age is consistent with the death, in August 1997, of Jeanne Calment in France—at 122, the longest well-documented life on record. The number 120, or something close to it, comes from comparisons across species from fruit flies to Galapagos turtles. In almost every species, the oldest age observed is approximately six times the length of time from birth to maturity. In the human case, this argues for a span of 108 or 120 years, assuming that the age of complete biological maturity is eighteen to twenty years. On the other hand, many scientists now feel that it is unlikely that there is any fixed life span limit.

More conservative predictions come from statisticians and mathematical demographers who focus not on the maximum age to which a person can live (which may or may not be fixed) but on the *average* age at death of the entire population. They estimate that average life expectancy at birth in the United States (now about seventy-six years) will reach eighty-three years by the year 2050 and that the practical upper limit of average human life expectancy may not be much more than that. Several lines of research lead them to this conclusion. First, as actuaries from the Social Security Administration point out, we have already experienced the great gains conferred by the widespread use of antibiotic drugs against infectious diseases; little more can be expected from this source. Second, further progress in preventing or deferring the onset of heart attacks, strokes, and cancer will be slower—and these are the major causes of death among older men and women.

Furthermore, some experts believe that even prevention or cure of cancer and heart disease would fail to take us beyond the eighty-five-year limit. Why? Because it has been observed that beginning at age twenty, human death rates for each decade are twice that of the preceding ten-year period. The same applies to regular increases in death rates among zoo animals and pets that are protected from the hazards of life in the wild. If this regularity reflects some unchanging law of nature, cutting out later life illness may not be a meaningful factor in lengthening life.

To understand the combined magnitude of these changes in life expectancy, let us think of the total population of our country as divided into five-year age groups. We begin with males and females just born, zero to four years of age, then those five to nine, ten to fourteen, and so on to the oldest old. The number of people, male and female, in each of these age groups is known. Those numbers can be represented visually by means of a bar chart, in which the length of each horizontal bar shows the millions of people in each age group, males on the left and females on the right, in each age group.

When such a chart is drawn for the years before 1900, it is shaped like a triangle or a pyramid, with the greatest numbers at the youngest ages and fewer people in each older age group (figure 1,

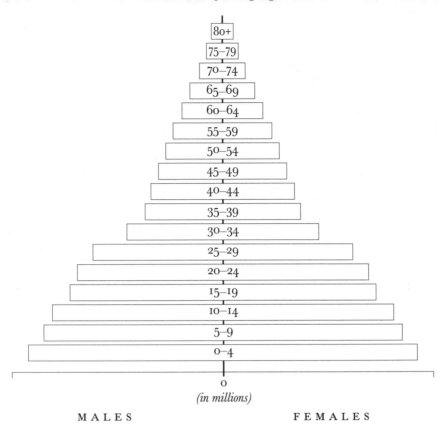

80+
75–79
70–74
65–69
60–64
55–59
50–54
45–49
40–44
35–39
30–34
25–29
20–24
15–19
10–14
5–9
0–4

0

(in millions)

MALES FEMALES

Figure 1. United States in 1900

from Olshansky, 1997). But the present and the future pattern, at least for the United States and other technologically advanced countries, is very different—more like a slightly lopsided rectangle or squat pillar than a pyramid (figure 2, from Olshansky, 1997). The rectangular shape means that infant mortality is very low, that the infectious diseases of childhood are greatly reduced, and that the impact of chronic diseases is postponed to old age. Substantial reductions in the length of the bars occur only after age sixty-five. The lopsided shape of the bars, especially after age sixty-five, shows the longer survival of women than men. Infants born in 1992 will live, on the average, to age seventy-six, but the women will live seven years longer than the men.

Not only are there more older people in our society than ever

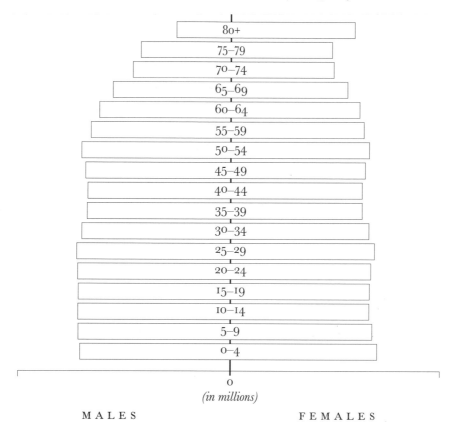

80+	
75–79	
70–74	
65–69	
60–64	
55–59	
50–54	
45–49	
40–44	
35–39	
30–34	
25–29	
20–24	
15–19	
10–14	
5–9	
0–4	

0

(in millions)

MALES   FEMALES

Figure 2. United States in the 21st Century

before, but those seniors are different than they used to be. The eminent gerontologist Bernice Neugarten first suggested that older people be divided into two groups, the "young-old," who are about age sixty-five to seventy-four, generally well and highly functional; and the "old-old," those over age seventy-five, who are much more likely to be frail. This latter group has also been referred to as in the "last quarter" of life. The old-old are by far the fastest-growing subset of the aging population. Of all individuals over age sixty-five in the United States in 1900, only 4 percent were over age eighty-five. Today, that proportion has reached over 10 percent, and continues to grow.

Another major change within the elderly population has been the emergence of a striking preponderance of women. The death rates for older men was only 5 percent higher than that for women in the year 1900. But in 1992, the death rate for women over age sixty-five was 23 percent lower than the corresponding rate for men. As mentioned previously, women aged sixty-five have an average of nineteen years of life expectancy as compared to fifteen years for similarly aged men. And life expectancy at birth for women has now reached seven years greater than that for men. Among those over the age of eighty-five, there are now five women for every two men. Aging in America has become, in many ways, a women's issue.

And there are several other key distinctions between today's and yesterday's elderly. In the past, older Americans were generally foreign born, spoke primarily foreign languages, had little education, and no access to high-quality health care. Today's and certainly tomorrow's older individuals generally have more education, greater access to health care, improved sanitary conditions, and greater financial worth than past generations of seniors had. A highly respected demographer, Samuel Preston, estimates in his book *The Oldest Old* that the proportion of individuals aged eighty-five to eighty-nine with seven or fewer years of education was greater than 60 percent in 1980, and will fall to as low as 10 to 15 percent by the year 2015. These improvements have resulted in a rapid increase in older people's ability to function, an issue we discuss in the next chapter on the myths of aging.

CHAPTER ONE

BREAKING DOWN THE MYTHS OF AGING

T HE TOPIC OF aging is durably encapsulated in a layer of myths in our society. And, like most myths, the ones about aging include a confusing blend of truth and fancy. We have compressed six of the most familiar of the aging myths into single-sentence assertions—frequently heard, usually with some link to reality, but always (thankfully) in significant conflict with recent scientific data.

> MYTH #1: To be old is to be sick.
>
> MYTH #2: You can't teach an old dog new tricks.
>
> MYTH #3: The horse is out of the barn.
>
> MYTH #4: The secret to successful aging is to choose your parents wisely.
>
> MYTH #5: The lights may be on, but the voltage is low.
>
> MYTH #6: The elderly don't pull their own weight.

Contrasting these myths with scientific fact leads to the conclusion that our society is in persistent denial of some important truths about aging. Our perceptions about the elderly fail to keep pace with the dramatic changes in their actual status. We view the aged as sick, demented, frail, weak, disabled, powerless, sexless, passive, alone, unhappy, and unable to learn—in short, a rapidly growing mass of irreversibly ill, irretrievable older Americans. To sum up, the elderly are depicted as a figurative ball and chain holding back an otherwise spry collective society. While this image is far from true, evidence that the bias persists is everywhere around us. Media attention to the elderly continues to be focused on their frailty, occasionally interspersed, in recent years, by equally unrealistic presentations of improbably youthful elders. Gerontologists, an important group of scholars which has become prominent during the last few decades, have been as much a part of the problem as the solution. Their literature has been preoccupied with concerns about frailty, nursing home admissions, and the social and health care needs of multiply impaired elders.

That we as a society are obsessed with the negative rather than the positive aspect of aging is not a new observation. Robert Butler, a pioneering gerontologist and geriatrician who was founding director of the National Institute on Aging and established the United States's first formal Department of Geriatric Medicine at Mount Sinai Medical Center in New York, coined the term "ageism" in his Pulitzer Prize-winning book *Growing Old in America—Why Survive?* in 1975. Butler saw ageism as similar to racism and sexism—a negative view of a group, and a view divorced from reality. More recently Betty Friedan, a leading architect of the women's movement, wrote about the mystique that surrounds aging in America, and our obsession with "the problem of aging." The persistence of the negative, mythic view of older persons as an unproductive burden has been underlined in recent congressional debates as to whether America can "afford the elderly." Ken Dychtwald, founder and CEO of Age Wave, Inc., has consistently sounded the call for a realistic view of aging and of older persons, exhorting American corporations to become more responsive to elders' needs.

. . .

Most of us resist replacing myth-based beliefs with science-based conclusions. It involves letting go of something previously ingrained in order to make way for the newly demonstrated facts. Learning something new requires "unlearning" something old and perhaps deeply rooted. Acknowledging the truth about aging in America is critical, however, if we are to move ahead toward successful aging as individuals and as a society. In order to make use of the new scientific knowledge and experience its benefits in our daily lives, we must first "unlearn" the myths of aging. Here we present each myth with a glimpse of the scientific evidence that corrects or contradicts it. In the following chapters of this book, we will explore that evidence in greater detail and discover its implications for how long, and how well, we live.

MYTH #1

"TO BE OLD IS TO BE SICK"

Ironically, myth #1 could be the title of many a gerontological text. Happily, though, the MacArthur Study and other important research has proved the statement false. Still, a central question regarding the status of the elderly is, "Just who is this new breed of seniors?" Are we facing an increased number of very sick old people, or is the new elder population healthier and more robust?

The first clue comes in the prevalence of diseases. Throughout the century there has been a shift in the patterns of sickness in the aging population. In the past, acute, infectious illness dominated. Today, chronic illnesses are far more prevalent. The most common ailments in today's elderly include the following: arthritis (which affects nearly half of all old people), hypertension and heart disease (which affect nearly a third), diabetes (11 percent), and disorders which influence communication such as hearing impairment (32 percent), cataracts (17 percent), and other forms of visual impairments including macular degeneration (9 percent). When you compare sixty-five- to seventy-four-year-old individuals in 1960 with those similarly aged in 1990, you find a dramatic reduction in the prevalence of three important precursors to chronic disease: high blood pressure, high cholesterol levels, and smoking. We also know that between 1982 and 1989, there were significant reductions in the prevalence of arthritis, arteriosclerosis (hardening of the arteries), dementia, hypertension, stroke and emphysema (chronic lung disease), as well as a dramatic decrease in the average number of diseases an older person has. And dental health has improved as well. The proportion of older individuals with dental disease so severe as to result in their having no teeth has dropped from 55 percent in 1957 to 34 percent in 1980, and is currently approaching 20 percent.

But what really matters is not the number or type of diseases one has, but how those problems impact on one's ability to function. For instance, if you are told that a white male is age seventy-five, your ability to predict his functional status is limited. Even if you are given details of his medical history, and learn he has a history of hypertension, diabetes, and has had a heart attack in the past, you still couldn't say whether he is sitting on the Supreme Court of the United States or in a nursing home!

There are two key ways to determine people's ability to remain independent. One is to assess their ability to manage their personal care. The personal care activities include basic functions, such as dressing, bathing, toileting, feeding oneself, transferring from bed to chair, and walking. The second category of activities is known as nonpersonal care. These are tasks such as preparing meals, shopping, paying bills, using the telephone, cleaning the house, writing, and reading. A person is disabled or dependent when he or she cannot perform some of these usual activities without assistance. When you look at sixty-five-year-old American men, who have a total life expectancy of fifteen more years, the picture is a surprisingly positive one: twelve years are likely to be spent fully independent. By age eighty-five, the picture is more bleak: nearly half of the future years are spent inactive or dependent.

Life expectancy for women is substantially greater than that for men. At age sixty-five, women have almost nineteen years to live—four more than men of the same age. And for women, almost fourteen of those will be active, and five years dependent.

It is important to recognize that this dependency is not purely a function of physical impairments but represents, particularly in advanced age, a mixture of physical and cognitive impairment. Even at age eighty-five, women have a life expectancy advantage of nearly one and a half years over men and are likely to spend about half of the rest of their lives independent.

There are two general schools of thought regarding the implications of increased life expectancy on the overall health status of the aging population. One holds that the same advances in medical technology will produce not only longer life, but also less disease and disability in old age. This optimistic theory predicts a reduction in the incidence of nonfatal disorders such as arthritis, dementia, hearing impairment, diabetes, hypertension, and the like. It is known as the "compression of morbidity" theory—in a nutshell, it envisions prolonged active life and delayed disability for older people. A contrasting theory maintains just the opposite: that our population will become both older and sicker.

The optimistic theory may be likened to the tale of the "one-horse shay" by Oliver Wendell Holmes. Some sixty-five to seventy years ago, when one of us (RLK) was reluctantly attending the Fairbanks Elementary School in Detroit, students were required to memorize poetry. One of Robert's favorites was a long set of verses by Oliver Wendell Holmes entitled "The Deacon's Masterpiece or The Wonderful One-Horse Shay." (A shay was a two-wheeled buggy, usually fitted with a folding top. The word itself, shay, is a New England adaptation from the French *chaise*.)

The relevance of all this to gerontology becomes clear early in the poem. The deacon was exasperated with the tendency of horse-drawn carriages to wear out irregularly; one part or another would fail when the rest of the vehicle was still in prime condition. He promised to build a shay in which every part was equally strong and durable, so that it would not be subject to the usual breakdowns of one or another part. And he was marvelously successful. The shay showed no sign of aging whatsoever until the first day of its 101st year, when it suddenly, instantly, and mysteriously turned to dust. The poem concludes with a line that stays in memory after all the intervening years. It is the poet's challenge to those who find the story difficult to believe. Since every part of the shay was equally durable, collapse of all had to come at the same moment: "End of the wonderful one-hoss shay; logic is logic; that's all I say."

The second, more negative theory—in which older people become sicker and more dependent with increasing age—is losing favor. MacArthur Studies and other research show us that older people are much more likely to age well than to become decrepit and dependent. The fact is, relatively few elderly people live in nursing homes. Only 5.2 percent of older people reside in such institutions, a figure which declined significantly from the 6.3 percent found in a 1982 survey. Furthermore, most older Americans are free of disabilities. Of those aged sixty-five to seventy-four in 1994, a full 89 percent report no disability whatsoever. While the proportion of elderly who are fully functioning and robust declines with advancing age, between the age of seventy-five to eighty-four, 73 percent still report no disability, and even after age eighty-five, 40 percent of the population is fully functional.

Between 1982 and 1994, the proportion of the population over age sixty-five that reported any disability fell from 24.9 percent to 21.3 percent, a meaningful reduction. And another statistic really sends the message home: in the United States today there are 1.4 million fewer disabled older people than there would be had the status of the elderly not improved since 1982. Furthermore, many studies show that the reduction in disability among older people appears to be accelerating. This is true at all ages, even among those over age ninety-five.

And so, the optimistic vision of aging seems to hold true—and the fact that the elderly population is relatively healthy and independent bears on the future of social policies for older people. It has important implications for issues as broad as establishing the proper eligibility age for Social Security benefits, and projecting the likely future expenses of federal health care programs including Medicare and Medicaid. Furthermore, beyond social policy implications, the greater our understanding of disability trends, the greater, in turn, will be our insights into the degree of biological change in our aging population. Disability in older people results from three key factors: 1) the impact of disease, or more commonly, many diseases at once; 2) lifestyle factors, such as exercise and diet, which directly influence physical fitness and risk of disease; and 3) the biological changes that occur with advancing age—formally known as senescence. It is not clear whether the reduction in the incidence of many chronic diseases—and the reduction in many risk factors for those diseases—is connected to a more general slowdown in the rate of physical aging. There is increasing evidence that the rate of physical aging is not, as we once believed, determined by genes alone. Lifestyle factors—which can be changed—have powerful influence as well. We will discuss this in much greater detail later in the book, but it's a very empowering notion to keep in mind. We can, and should, take some responsibility for the way in which we grow older.

So far, we have been focusing on objective information about older people's ability to function. But another important issue is how older people *perceive* their own health status. Again, we are optimistic. Research finds that older people have a quite positive view of their own health. In one major study, older people were asked to rate their health as excellent, very good, good, fair, or poor. In 1994, 39 percent of individuals over the age of sixty-five viewed their health as very good or excellent, while only 29 percent considered their health to be fair or poor. Even among those over age eighty-five, 31 percent considered themselves to be in very good or excellent health, while 36 percent viewed themselves as in poor health. Men and women were equally positive, but there were some racial differences—for instance, older African Americans were more likely than Caucasians to rate their health as poor. In general, however, a growing body of evidence shows that older people perceive themselves as healthy, even in the face of real physical problems. Why the occasional dissonance between objective measures of health and people's perceptions of it? It may reflect a remarkably successful adaptation to disability. Despite society's view of older persons as frail and in poor health, older people simply don't share that view, even when they have objective evidence of disability.

In sum, decades of research clearly debunk the myth that to be old in America is to be sick and frail. Older Americans are generally healthy. Even in advanced old age, an overwhelming majority of the elderly population have little functional disability, and the proportion that is disabled is being whittled away over time. We are delighted to observe increasing momentum toward the emergence of a physically and cognitively fit, nondisabled, active elderly population. The combination of longer life and less illness is adding life to years as well as years to life.

At the same time, as a result of the MacArthur Foundation Studies of Aging in America and other research, we now can identify the lifestyle and personality factors that boost the chance of aging successfully. This book discusses strategies to reduce one's risk of disease and disability, and to maintain physical and mental function. Our main message is that we can have a dramatic impact on our own success or failure in aging. Far more than is usually assumed, successful aging is in our own hands. What we can do for ourselves, however, depends partly on the opportunities and constraints that are presented to us as we age—in short, on the attitudes and expectations of others toward older people, and on policies of the larger society of which we are a part.

MYTH #2

"YOU CAN'T TEACH AN OLD DOG NEW TRICKS"

The pervasive belief among young and old that the elderly cannot sharpen or broaden their minds creates a disturbing cycle of mental inactivity and decay. Certainly, the less people are challenged, the less they can perform. But research shows that older people can, and do, learn new things—and they learn them well. True, the limits of learning, and especially the pace of learning, are more restricted in age than in youth. And the conditions for successful learning are different for older people than for the young. The trouble is, our institutions of learning—schools and work organizations—have not yet adapted to these age differences. One result is that the myth about older people's capacity to grow and learn becomes further entrenched.

MacArthur research on mental function in old age is also encouraging. First of all, the fears of age-related loss are often exaggerated. Older people have become so sensitized to the threat of Alzheimer's disease that every forgotten name or misplaced key ring strikes fear. Alzheimer's is indeed a terrible disease, both for those afflicted and their caregivers. But current estimates are that no more than 10 percent of all elderly people, aged sixty-five to one hundred or more, are Alzheimer's patients. In fact, even among those aged seventy-four to eighty-one, a full half show no mental decline whatsoever over the following seven years. Ninety-five percent of older people live in the community at large; only 5 percent are in nursing homes. And that small percentage has been decreasing since 1982! The MacArthur Studies have added to our understanding of the factors that maintain high mental function. As we discuss in chapter 8, three key features predict strong mental function in old age: 1) regular physical activity; 2) a strong social support system; and 3) belief in one's ability to handle what life has to offer. Happily, all three can be initiated or increased, even in later life.

Older Men and Women Can and Do Learn New Things

Research has demonstrated the remarkable and enduring capacity of the aged brain to make new connections, absorb new data, and thus acquire new skills. In one experiment, older people who showed a decline in two important cognitive functions, inductive reasoning and spatial orientation, participated in five training sessions designed to improve these functions. The improvements were significant, and permanent. The same can be said of short-term memory among older men and women. Before training sessions, older people were able to recall fewer than five words from a randomly presented long list. After training, they were able to recall almost fifteen words. (In chapter 8, we go into this in more detail.) As consumers, older people learn to use household appliances that were unknown in their youth—food processors, microwave ovens, automated bank teller machines, and even "user-friendly" VCRs (video cassette recorders). Secretaries who learned their craft on manual typewriters make the transition to electric machines and then to word processors and computers.

The stereotype in organizations is that older people oppose innovation while younger ones urge it—the stereotypical old fogies versus the young Turks. But in fact, corporate battles often involve young fogies and old Turks! Intimate knowledge of a given organization, the security that often comes with long tenure and, ultimately, the freedom that accompanies impending retirement combine to yield significant advantages to older people in the workplace. Specifically, elders may have an innovative advantage that compensates for (or even exceeds) the flexibility of youth.

Some Aspects of Learning Are More Limited in Age

Science confirms what all of us have observed; young people

tend to have sharper vision and better hearing than older people, their reaction time is quicker, and they outperform elders in terms of short-term memory. As a result, some kinds of learning, especially those that require perceptual speed, physical coordination, and muscular strength, become more difficult and ultimately impossible in old age. One of us (RLK) was, in his late teens, an aspiring gymnast. Robert mastered some modest feats, but the giant swing, in which the performer does a handstand on the high bar, was beyond his reach. Back then, he probably could have prevailed with a little extra training (and perhaps courage). At age eighty, the giant swing is beyond the realm of possibility. As we write this, however, we have before us a picture of the man who, as a senior Olympic competitor, holds the national record for pole vault. He is sixty-seven years old! So while there are certainly limits, there are limit-breakers as well.

What It Takes to Learn Changes with Age

While it is true that older people have, in general, weaker short-term memories than younger people, these deficits can be overcome with proper training. For instance, older people can significantly improve their short-term memory by making lists and training their memory with practice games. Admittedly, similarly trained young people do still better, but trained elders often do better than untrained young people.

There are many examples of ways in which older people can boost their performance when given the right opportunity for improvement. The key is for older people to develop at their own pace, and with respect for both their practical and emotional needs. One good example is the case of a large company that was converting to computer-controlled operation of a decentralized staff. They soon found that older workers were relatively slow, and reluctant to adapt to the new procedures. Young people, already computer proficient, were assigned as coaches, but the difficulties continued. In time, older clerks were seen staying at their desks beyond the usual working hours, in order to practice in relative privacy and at their own pace. And indeed, their performance improved significantly. This episode illustrates several of the key requirements for learning new skills in old age. It is critical that older people be able to 1) work at their own pace; 2) practice new skills; and 3) avoid the embarrassment so common among older people when they cannot keep up to speed with their younger counterparts. From childhood, we become accustomed to older people teaching those who are younger. It is often difficult for older people to accept the reversal of roles in which the young become the mentors.

Teaching Institutions Haven't Adapted to Learning Needs

When it comes to learning, our society is still age-graded. Times have changed, the need for lifelong learning and relearning has increased, but our institutions have not caught up with the new realities. They operate as if life consisted of three compartmentalized periods—education, work, and retirement, in that order.

There was a time when that was adequate. The traditional skills of reading, writing, and arithmetic were sufficient for many jobs. More specific skills, once learned, were practiced for the rest of one's working life. That time is long gone. Technological change means that most people will need to learn several new jobs in the course of their working lives. We now know that the capacity to learn is lifelong. The next step will be to create the conditions under which lifelong learning can be nurtured and achieved.

MYTH #3

"THE HORSE IS OUT OF THE BARN"

We've all heard the claims of lifelong smokers that there's "no point stopping now"—the damage is already done and the habit permanently ingrained. This is an easy way out, but far from the truth. It's time to dispel the false and discouraging claim that old age is too late for efforts to reduce risk and promote health. Many older persons believe that after decades of risky behavior—overindulgence in alcohol and fat-laden food, lack of exercise, and so on—there is no point changing. They feel that what they have lost is gone forever and cannot be recovered, or they deny that their habits are dangerous in the first place. Many consider age-related changes irreversible, and hold no hope for either recovering lost function or lessening their risks of developing diseases. Fortunately, they are mistaken. Not only can we recover much lost function and decrease risk, but in some cases we can actually increase function beyond our prior level.

Mark Twain amused his audiences by reversing the relationship between health and bad habits. He told a story about an elderly woman whose doctor, after careful examination, informed her that she would have to quit smoking, drinking, and gorging herself on rich food.

"But doctor," she protested, "I have never done any of those things in my life!"

At this point, Twain looked out at the audience. There was a moment of silence, he shook his white head sadly, and pronounced the grim verdict: "There you are. There was nothing to be done. She had neglected her habits!"

Certainly, it's better to start healthy habits early and sustain them for a lifetime. But for those who have strayed—that is, most people!—nature is remarkably forgiving. Research shows that it is almost never too late to begin healthy habits such as smoking cessation, sensible diet, exercise, and the like. And even more important, it is never too late to benefit from those changes. Making these changes can mark the transition from the risky state we call "usual aging" to the goal we all share: "successful aging"—growing old with good health, strength, and vitality.

We're not, however, promoting a fantastical fountain of youth. Attempts at rejuvenation are probably as old as aging itself. Early in this century one of the more interesting (though ineffective) attempts involved injections of extracts of tiger testes. Though many anti-aging remedies and nostrums continue to be commercially available, most have little to offer or are, at best, of unproven value. We discuss these in greater detail in chapter 9. Despite the lack of proven "rejuvenators," however, there are many ways in which older people can recover function and decrease the risk of disease or disability. Perhaps the greatest anti-aging "potion" is good old-fashioned clean living.

Cigarette Smoking

Everyone knows that smoking is bad for the health. But we've heard it so often, and for so long, it often falls on deaf ears. Cigarette smoking and other tobacco use increases the risk of lung cancer and other lung diseases, coronary heart disease, stroke, and other life-threatening illnesses. A person who smokes a pack of cigarettes a day is four times more likely than a nonsmoker to have coronary heart disease. Even a person who smokes less than half a pack a day is twice as likely to have coronary heart disease as a nonsmoker. That's the bad news.

The good news is that the risk of heart disease begins to fall almost as soon as you quit smoking—no matter how long you've smoked. Within a few months, smokers who have managed to quit begin to reap the benefits. In five years, an ex-smoker is not much more likely to have heart disease than a person who has never smoked! That's only part of the good news about smoking and heart disease. The rest of it is that the good effects of quitting smoking hold regardless of age, the number of years one smokes, or how heavy the smoking habit.

Like heart disease, the risk of stroke drops quickly when cigarette smoking stops. We know that among people aged thirty-four to fifty-five, those who stopped smoking within the past two to four years were no more at risk for stroke than those who had never smoked at all.

Lung disease, especially lung cancer and emphysema, is perhaps the main fear of cigarette smokers. In this case, too, the research is encouraging to former smokers and should spur those who are planning to stop. As with heart disease, the risk of lung cancer begins to fall when smoking stops, although much more slowly. It takes at least fifteen years after quitting for a smoker's risk of lung cancer to become as low as that of a lifetime nonsmoker. But the good news remains; when you quit, your lungs begin to heal and the risk of lung disease begins to drop. That holds for people of all ages.

Being overweight and eating too much of the wrong things is like smoking in some ways. Psychologists call these activities oral gratification—and like smoking, eating habits are hard to change. Unfortunately, overeating is like smoking in another way: it increases the risk of many diseases. Several factors fit together like a puzzle and conspire to raise the risk of disease: eating too many calories, eating too much fat, and becoming obese. All of these—independently and as a group—may raise the risk of heart disease as well as certain cancers.

Syndrome X

Researchers have identified a new condition known as Syndrome X, in which a cluster of risk factors together raise the risk of heart attack and premature death. These factors include high blood sugar and insulin levels (the so-called pseudodiabetes of aging); high blood pressure; and increases in blood fats like cholesterol and triglycerides, which accompany the pot-bellied obesity so common in middle-aged and elderly people (especially men). But the good news for people with Syndrome X is that the increased risk of heart disease is related to their weight, not their age. When their weight drops and stays down, so do the risk factors for heart disease. These results hold in old age. When obese middle-aged and older men lose 10 percent of their body weight, they reduce their risk factors significantly. In one study, older men lost less weight than younger ones, but interestingly, they did almost as well in reducing their risk of disease.

High Blood Pressure

High blood pressure, especially the systolic blood pressure (the higher of the two numbers in your blood pressure reading), is an important risk factor for heart disease and stroke. In the United States and other similarly prosperous countries, systolic blood pressure generally rises with age. In fact, the increase in blood pressure is so common that it is often taken for granted, and considered the inevitable result of "normal" aging. But in developed countries, not *all* older people show increases in blood pressure; and on the flip side of the coin, in less-advantaged countries, where people eat less meat, more grains and vegetables, and keep physically active, blood pressure tends *not* to rise with age.

Diet and exercise tend to reduce blood pressure, but they are not failproof. Some people do neither, and have low blood pressure. And others do both, but are unable to lower their blood pressure to an acceptable level. In a reversal from previous practice, such older individuals are now commonly advised to take medication to get their blood pressure under control. But many older people resist drug treatment, arguing that they have tolerated their hypertension well for many years, and that certainly the damage is already done. But we now know that treatment of systolic hypertension is safe, inexpensive, and lowers risk. One large study, in which all the participants were over the age of sixty and some were over eighty, showed that drug treatments for high blood pressure reduced the risk of stroke by more than a third and the risk of heart attacks by more than a quarter. The horse may have been headed out of the barn, but some good rope tricks lured it back in.

Physical Fitness

"Doc, I've been a couch potato for so many years, I can't possibly get back in shape" is a common refrain in my (JWR) office. Physical function does indeed decrease with age, especially in the realm of the upper limits of physical performance. The best race times of elderly marathon runners and master swimmers do not equal those of similarly trained young athletes (nor of their own performance in the days of their youth). Nerve function, heart capacity, kidney function, breathing capacity, and maximum work rate all show age-related reductions. Vision and hearing, muscle mass, and strength show similar age-related patterns. That's the bad news. But set against this tale of diminishing capacities are three reassuring facts.

First, the aged body is more than able to meet the demands of everyday life. Losses in elite athletic ability do not create handicaps for most activities.

Second, most age-related reductions in physical performance are avoidable and many are reversible. They are often the cumulative result of lifestyle—what we do with our bodies and what we take into them—rather than the result of aging itself. Years of cigarette smoking, excessive use of alcohol, too little exercise and too much food, especially fats and sugars, do physical damage that is often wrongly attributed to age.

The facts are that exercise dramatically increases physical fitness, muscle size, and strength in older individuals. Besides rejuvenating muscles, resistance exercises (pumping iron) also enhance bone strength, limiting the risk of osteoporosis and fractures of the hip, spine, and wrist. Exercise also improves balance, thereby decreasing the risk of falling, a common and life-threatening problem in older persons. And as we discuss in detail in chapter 7, the MacArthur Studies now show that physical exercise is just the first of several ways to maintain one's physical abilities. It turns out that active mental stimulation, and keeping up relationships with friends and relatives, also helps promote physical ability. For instance, many people are surprised to learn that frequent emotional support (listening, encouragement, cheering up, understanding, and so on) is associated with improved physical function in old age. This is just one of countless connections between mind and body—mental vigor and physical well-being—that are seen in the aging process. A healthy physical and emotional lifestyle seems to be of even greater value to older people than younger ones. It's never too late to start.

"THE SECRET TO SUCCESSFUL AGING IS TO CHOOSE YOUR PARENTS WISELY"

People commonly assume that genes (or heredity) account for the rate at which one's body functions decline with advancing age. And it's not hard to find examples to support that assumption—families in which everyone seems to live past ninety or not make it to age sixty-five. True, there is a meaningful connection between genetics and aging. For instance, it has long been recognized that the length of life of nonidentical twins varies much more than that of identical twins. But while the role of genetics in aging is important, it has been tremendously overstated. A common error is to assume that one's genetic predisposition is equivalent to genetic "control" of life expectancy, and that we are all preprogrammed for a given duration of life. Our MacArthur twin studies leave very substantial room for factors *other* than genetics in determining life expectancy.

When considering what factors promote long life, it is essential to distinguish familial habits and experiences from genes. Members of a family may share many characteristics as they grow old, but this should not be misinterpreted as evidence for a pure genetic role in aging. It is possible that these similarities are related more to common environmental conditions, such as diet, which are shared by family members. Not everything that runs in families is genetic. For example, apple pie recipes, though passed from generation to generation, are clearly not genetically determined. But the contents of those apple pies, and all other foods shared by families, have a meaningful impact on the health of all family members—their weight, blood sugar levels, you name it.

Regardless of our genes, we as individuals can play an important role in how successfully we age. Just how big a role can we play? That depends on the balance between the influence of genes and environment. Let's take a look at the ways in which heredity does—and does not—play an important role in the three key components of successful aging: 1) avoiding disease and disability; 2) maintaining high mental and physical function; and 3) continuing to engage actively in life, through productivity and strong interpersonal relationships.

The strongest influence of heredity on aging relates to genetic diseases that can shorten life, such as numerous forms of cancer and familial high cholesterol syndromes (which lead to heart disease). Certainly, it would behoove us to choose parents who don't carry genes for these diseases. Would that it were so easy. Still, however, heredity is not as powerful a player as many assume. For all but the most strongly determined genetic diseases, such as Huntington's disease, MacArthur Studies show that the environment and lifestyle have a powerful impact on the likelihood of actually developing the disorder. This is wonderful news for individuals with strong family histories of some cancers, heart disease, hypertension, rheumatoid arthritis, and many other conditions. We now know that diet, exercise, and even medications may delay, or completely eliminate, the emergence of the disease. Genes play a key role in promoting disease, but they are certainly less than half the story.

What about the role of genetics on mental and physical function, the second important component of successful aging? In this arena, MacArthur research has shown that heredity is *less* important than environment and lifestyle. A major study of Swedish twins that was part of the MacArthur Research Program on Successful Aging shed light on the factors that influence the physiological changes that occur with advancing age. By studying both identical and nonidentical twins who were raised apart, researchers were able to tease apart the relative importance of heredity and environment on mental and physical changes with age. The bottom line is very clear: with rare exceptions, only about 30 percent of physical aging can be blamed on the genes. Additional studies of Swedish twins over the age of 80 show that only about half of the changes in mental function with aging are genetic. This leaves substantial room for a healthy lifestyle to protect the mind and body. And better yet, as we grow older, genetics becomes *less* important, and environment becomes *more* important. The likelihood of being fat, having hypertension, high cholesterol and triglyceride levels, and the rate at which one's lung function declines with advancing age are, by and large, largely *not* inherited. These risks are due to environmental or lifestyle factors. How we live, and where we live, has the most profound impact on age-related changes in the function of many organs throughout the body, including the heart, immune system, lung, bones, brain, and kidneys. We will discuss these important findings in greater detail in chapters 5–8.

The third component of successful aging, continuing active engagement with life, is for the most part not inherited. While certain personality traits may be, in part, heritable—the maintenance of good health certainly enhances the likelihood of remaining active and engaged in life—one's degree of vitality and interpersonal connection late in life is largely determined by *nongenetic* factors.

These findings are exceptionally optimistic and shatter the myth that our course in old age is predetermined. MacArthur research provides very strong scientific evidence that we are, in large part, responsible for our own old age. We have the powerful capacity to enhance our chance of maintaining high mental and physical ability as we grow older. Throughout this book, we will show you just how that can be accomplished.

MYTH #5

"THE LIGHTS MAY BE ON, BUT THE VOLTAGE IS LOW"

This metaphorical assertion has at least three implications about aging—all negative and none accurate. The myth suggests that older people suffer from inadequate physical and mental abilities. And the electrical metaphor hints that older men and women are sexless, or at least uninterested in sex (and, in the case of men, unable to perform adequately regardless of interest). MacArthur research shows that while there is some modicum of truth to these beliefs, they're far more fiction than fact. Let's sift out the facts.

Sexuality in Old Age

At the time of this writing, a popular TV beverage commercial pokes fun at a silver-haired couple engaged in passionate foreplay on the living room couch. The image is presented as absurd, and a humorous reference is made to the parents (supposedly 100-plus years old) being home. Apparently, the age-old assumption that sexual interest and activity in later life are rare and inappropriate is still in full force. These stereotypical images are examples of what psychologists call "pluralistic ignorance"—that is, most people as private individuals know the image is false, but remain silent on the subject because they think that others see it as true.

We remind ourselves that myths do contain some truth. Sexual activity *does* tend to decrease in old age. However, there are tremendous individual differences in this intimate aspect of life. We know also that these differences are determined in part by cultural norms, by health or illness, and by the availability of sexual or romantic partners. When it comes to sexual activity, as in so many other aspects of aging, chronological age itself is not the critical factor. In men, the decline in testosterone with age is highly variable and linked only loosely with sexual performance.

Certainly there are older people who have lost interest in sex and are glad to be done with it. When Sophocles, the great tragic poet of ancient Greece, was in his eighties, he was asked rather delicately whether, at his advanced age, he "had yet any acquaintance with Venus." "Heavens forbid!" the sage is said to have replied, "I thank the gods that I am finally rid of that tyranny."

Had surveys been conducted in the Greece of 400 B.C., it is unlikely that all of his elderly countrymen (and women) would have agreed with him. Certainly it is not the dominant view of older men and women in the United States today. There is a gradual decline in sexual interest and ability beginning around the age of fifty. However, this decline has many causes besides age itself, including certain chronic diseases and the medications with which they are treated. Diabetes, heart disease, and hypertension are perhaps the most frequent impediments to sexual function, especially for men.

At least since the famous Kinsey report in 1953, there have been occasional attempts to put numbers to the question of sexual activity in old age. One important early study found that at age sixty-eight, about 70 percent of men were sexually active on a regular basis. At age seventy-eight, however, the percentage dropped to about 25 percent of men. In addition to age itself, health status was the major factor in determining the frequency of sexual activity among men. For older women, however, regularity of sexual activity depends primarily on the availability of an appropriate partner. If this study were repeated today, the substantial improvements in health among older people and the changes in social norms that have occurred during the past two decades would likely yield evidence of even greater interest and participation in sex in later life.

Finally, our wish list for research on this important subject includes a distinction between the sex act itself and the many other forms of physical intimacy. The basic human need for affectionate physical contact, which is apparent even in newborn infants, persists throughout life. The voltage is never too low for that—in fact, it may help keep the lights on.

MYTH #6

"THE ELDERLY DON'T PULL THEIR OWN WEIGHT"

The widespread belief that older people are relatively unproductive in society is wrong and unjust in three ways: 1) the measures of performance are wrong; our society doesn't count a great deal of productive activity; 2) the playing field is not level; older men and women aren't given an equal chance for paying jobs; and 3) millions of older people are ready, willing, and able to increase their productivity, paid and voluntary. Let's look at the facts that bear on each of these claims.

The Measures Are Wrong

The accusation that older people are burdens rather than contributors to society is heard in many places, from the halls of Congress to the living rooms of overworked young men and women. The unstated assumptions are that everybody who works for pay is pulling his or her weight, and that everyone who does not work for pay is a burden.

Both assumptions are wrong. Some people who are paid do little or nothing useful, and some are paid to do things that are damaging—writing advertisements for cigarettes, for example. It is ironic and misleading, as well as unfair, that such things are counted as productive, while raising children, maintaining a household, taking care of an ill or disabled family member, or working as a volunteer in a hospital or church are considered unproductive (or at least not "counted" as productive). While it is important to distinguish between paid and unpaid work, it is wrong to omit unpaid productive work from our national accounting. As people age, and especially as they retire from paid work, their continuing productive activities are increasingly unpaid. Our national statistics thus ignore a great deal of productive activity, a great deal of what keeps our society functioning.

Almost all older men and women are productive in this larger sense. One-third work for pay and one-third work as volunteers in churches, hospitals, and other organizations. Others provide informal, much-needed assistance to family members, friends, and neighbors. It would take more than three million paid caregivers, working full time, to provide that assistance to sick and disabled people!

In 1997, a national campaign was mounted to increase volunteerism in America. The president and several ex-presidents spoke of the country's need for voluntary activity and urged people to contribute as volunteers. We propose one way of making it more attractive to volunteer: start counting voluntary work as productive. The ways we measure productive activity are broken; fix them!

The Playing Field Is Not Level

Older men and women aren't given an equal chance for paid employment. Retirement used to be compulsory. When you reached the ages of fifty-five or sixty or sixty-five, you had to retire. While it is now illegal to force people to retire solely because of their age, downsizing, corporate mergers, and other organizational changes affect older people disproportionately. For many people retirement, while not legally compelled, is nevertheless involuntary.

In addition to the stick of involuntary retirement, there is the carrot of pension entitlements, both private and through Social Security. These make retirement attractive or, for some, downright irresistible. We should remember, however, that the reasons for creating Social Security in the first place were not only to prevent poverty in old age but also to make way for youth. In an economy plagued by unemployment, getting older workers out of the labor force was an attractive idea. It exchanged unwanted joblessness among younger people for a more acceptable kind of joblessness (retirement) at the other end of the age range. In combination, both public and private policies urge older people to retire and we then blame them for doing so.

Older people who want to continue working beyond the usual retirement age see the inflexibility of employers as the main obstacle. Many of those who are still working and would like to continue with the same employer want fewer hours, a change in work content, or greater flexibility in scheduling. Ninety percent of those who want such changes, however, say that their employers will not accommodate them. Older people who are seeking new jobs report that companies are reluctant to hire older workers. Many employers seem to believe, mistakenly, that older workers are less productive, more often absent, or are liabilities in some other respect. When it comes to job-hunting by older people, the playing field has yet to be leveled.

They Are Ready, Willing, and Able

When Old Age and Survivors Insurance (OASI) was first enacted, most people did not live to the legal retirement age of sixty-five years. Most of those who did, it was assumed, would be neither willing nor able to work. Since the early twentieth century, life expectancy has greatly increased and the health of older people has greatly improved. Although some are not able to work and some do not wish to work, there are millions of older men and women who are ready, willing, and able to work. Among nonworkers aged fifty to fifty-nine, almost half would prefer to work, and among those sixty to sixty-four, more than one-third agree. Companies that have emphasized the recruitment and retention of older workers confirm that older employees meet or surpass expectations, often bringing the added value of increased insight and experience to the work environment.

CHAPTER TWO

THE STRUCTURE OF SUCCESSFUL AGING

S ATCHEL PAIGE, BASEBALL'S legendary, indestructible African-American pitcher, was as famous for his fast answers as for his fastball. He began pitching at the age of seventeen, and was for many years restricted to what was then called the Negro Baseball League. Born near the turn of the century, he was already a veteran at the pitcher's mound when the racial barrier was relaxed. However, the decades rolled by, and he continued to pitch. As he did so, Paige became purposefully vague about his age, a subject of increasing speculation among sportswriters. When one of them put the question bluntly—"How old *are* you?"—Paige gave him a classic answer: "How old would *you* be if you didn't know how old you was?"

The question—and Paige's answer—have as much to do with society's definitions and expectations of aging, and successful aging, as with Paige's own personal experience. By physical measures, at least, Paige was certainly aging successfully. But his wariness about coming clean with a hard number speaks volumes about our society's skepticism about competence in old age. What, after all, does it mean to "age successfully"? Does America think of aging per se as a bad thing, even when good things continue to develop—or emerge for the first time—with age? What, actually, is "success"?

A short time ago, one of us entered "success" into his computer as a keyword and was instantly rewarded with 2,670 entries on the subject. A quick scan of them revealed that "success" and "successful" are commonly used to indicate high income and wealth. That is not how we define success in this book. William James, the American philosopher and psychologist, said almost a century ago that "the squalid cash interpretation put on the word 'success' is our national disease." Successful aging does not refer to prosperity, although poverty certainly makes its attainment more difficult.

Roget's Thesaurus, that ultimate source of synonyms and phrases, gives us a broader definition of success. It tells us that to succeed is "to flourish, do well, be on top of the world, be on the crest of a wave." That brings us closer to the meaning we seek, but our concept of success connotes more than a happy outcome; it implies achievement rather than mere good luck. Being born to teethe on the proverbial silver spoon may be a sign of good fortune, but it does not indicate success. To succeed in something requires more than falling into it; it means having desired it, planned it, worked for it. All these factors are critical to our view of aging which, even in this era of human genetics, we regard as largely under the control of the individual. In short, successful aging is dependent upon individual choices and behaviors. It can be attained through individual choice and effort. Throughout this book, we will examine what successful aging consists of, and what each of us can do to achieve it.

DEFINING SUCCESSFUL AGING

Most people, when asked to distinguish between successful and unsuccessful aging, would think first of the difference between sickness and health. It is a good place to begin, but it is only a beginning.

For many years, gerontologists were concerned mainly with just that issue or, as they put it, with the distinction between pathologic and nonpathologic states. That view of aging has unacceptably narrow implications, however. It implies that, in the absence of some identifiable clinical disease or disability, all is well. It also implies that in the presence of disease, some kind of personal failure has occurred.

Certainly freedom from disease and disability is an important component of successful aging. All of us have experienced the life-greeting euphoria, usually all too brief, that comes with recovery from illness, even a severe case of flu. But absence of disease is not enough. A person who is not ill may nevertheless be at serious risk of illness or disability. And a person who is not at risk in those respects may nevertheless be living a lonely and inactive old age. Our definition of successful aging takes account of all these facts.

We therefore define successful aging as the ability to maintain three key behaviors or characteristics:

- low risk of disease and disease-related disability;
- high mental and physical function; and
- active engagement with life.

All three components are represented in figure 3. Each factor is important in itself, and to some extent independent of the others. Examples of this are all around us. For instance, Stephen Hawking, considered by many to be the greatest living physicist, has for years been severely disabled by amyotrophic lateral sclerosis, or Lou Gehrig's disease. He tells us that although his body is bound to a wheelchair, his mind is free to explore the limits of the universe. Mother Teresa's inspiring service to the poor of India continued in spite of her own physical infirmities. Franklin Roosevelt led the United States out of a great economic depression and through the greatest of wars, despite the crippling effects of poliomyelitis. We applaud such heroic achievements under conditions of physical

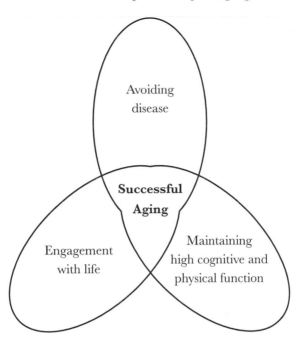

Figure 3. Components of Successful Aging

handicap, but we recognize also that freedom from disease and disability is a positive thing.

There is a kind of hierarchical ordering among the three components of successful aging. The absence of disease and disability makes it easier to maintain mental and physical function. And maintenance of mental and physical function in turn enables (but does not guarantee) active engagement with life. It is the *combination* of all three—avoidance of disease and disability, maintenance of cognitive and physical function, and sustained engagement with life—that represents the concept of successful aging most fully. Furthermore, each of these components of successful aging is itself a combination of factors. Avoiding disease and disability refers not only to the absence or presence of disease itself, but also to the absence or presence of *risk factors* for disease and disability. Maintaining a high level of overall functioning requires both physical and mental abilities, which are substantially independent of each other. And finally, these physical and mental capacities are only potentials for activity; they tell us what a person *can* do, but not what he or she actually *does*. Many older people, for many reasons, do much less than they are capable of doing. Successful aging goes beyond potential; it involves activity, which we have labeled "engagement with life." Active engagement with life takes many forms, but successful aging is most concerned with two—relationships with other people, and behavior that is productive. Not surprisingly, when asked their "secret" to aging well, many of the "successful agers" from the MacArthur Study echo the same refrain: "Just keep on going." It is this forward-looking, active engagement with life and with other human beings that is so critical to growing old *well*.

Now let us look more closely at each of the components of successful aging.

AVOIDING DISEASE AND DISABILITY

Modern medicine, of which we are all beneficiaries, has developed as an applied science of repair rather than prevention. In recent years, medical education has been moving slowly toward a more inclusive orientation, which emphasizes prevention as well as cure. However, the field of geriatrics has been much slower to make this shift, and public perceptions and attitudes have only started to move toward that larger, wellness-oriented view, and to accept its implications for daily life.

The very word "patient," which is what we call ourselves when we seek medical care, implies passivity rather than responsibility for our own health.

Of course, vulnerability to diseases and disabilities is not wholly under our control, nor is it likely to become so. Bad things indeed happen to good people and human life is, in part, subject to negative events that are neither predictable nor avoidable. But many illnesses and disabilities, especially the chronic diseases of old age, are preceded by signs of future problems. And too often, we—and our doctors—ignore those signs. Among these leading warning signs are modest increases in systolic blood pressure, abdominal fat, and blood sugar, and decreases in lung, kidney, and immune function. These changes, along with typical losses of bone density and muscle mass, constitute the syndrome of "usual aging," which we discuss in chapter 3. The bad news is that they are widespread—hence "usual." The good news is that they are caused, in large part, by extrinsic factors—how we live and what we eat—and therefore they are not our unavoidable destiny; they can be modified.

One of the main reasons we tend to ignore the warning signs of disease is that those signs can be silent or invisible. You don't "feel" high blood pressure until it makes you sick; you don't "feel" bone loss until you sustain a fracture; and so on. Furthermore, conventional medical practice tends to set standards for distinguishing between disease and its absence, ignoring the risky gray area in between the two. A blood pressure reading of 140/90 (systolic/diastolic) is the usual dividing line between hypertension and "normality." But nature is continuous, not dichotomous; with rare exceptions, people whose blood pressure exceeds the 140/90 level do not jump suddenly from normal to hypertensive. Their pattern over time would show gradual increases in blood pressure, through the so-called normal and high-normal range, until they finally reach the formal point of disease. Only then are they referred for treatment.

A preventive orientation would involve periodic monitoring and action, initially through diet and exercise, in response to modest increases in blood pressure—even in the range usually considered "normal." And the same would apply to other risk factors for chronic diseases in old age, such as gradual increases in cholesterol, blood sugar, and body weight.

Of course, prevention does not supplant surgical and medical remedies for disability and illness. Many older people with arthritis, for instance, who would once have been severely restricted in activity and mobility, are now enjoying pain-free, active lives because of successful hip replacement. In the 1930s the fatal hypertension of RLK's mother, like that of her mother before her, was called "essential" and uncontrollable. Any physician now seeing such patients can choose from an extensive armamentarium of drugs to bring their blood pressure down to less threatening levels.

MAINTAINING MENTAL AND PHYSICAL FUNCTION

Older people, like younger ones, want to be independent. This is the principal goal of many elders, and few issues strike greater fear than the prospect of depending on others for the most basic daily needs. Independence means continuing to live in one's own home, taking care of oneself, and carrying out the routines of daily life—dressing and washing, housework, shopping, and meal preparation. Especially in the United States, where many people live in single homes, where stores are concentrated in shopping malls, and public transportation is limited, living independently also means driving an automobile.

The ability to do all these things depends on maintaining physical and mental function, not necessarily at the level of elderly marathon runners and polymaths, but enough to carry on. Older men and women are therefore sensitive, often oversensitive, to any sign that they may be losing these functional capacities. Every lapse— misplaced car keys or a forgotten name—brings to mind the looming fear of Alzheimer's disease. But MacArthur research has three reassuring messages on the subject of maintaining function in old age: first, many of the fears about functional loss are exaggerated; second, much functional loss can be prevented; and third, many functional losses can be regained.

Exaggerated Fears

Consider just a few of the exaggerations. Alzheimer's disease is indeed a terrible condition, but it is not as common as many believe. A reasonable estimate is that 10 percent of people over the age of sixty-five are Alzheimer's patients; 90 percent of older people are not.

Furthermore, Alzheimer's disease is almost certainly not an all-or-nothing phenomenon. Even the characteristic "plaques and tangles" in the brains of Alzheimer's patients, which have long been considered the postmortem gold standard for diagnosis of the disease, are not infallible signs of its presence. They have been observed also in the brains of people who showed no symptoms of Alzheimer's. Pathology reports from the widely publicized Nun Study indicated that Sister Mary, who demonstrated superior cognitive ability until her death at age 101, had a high count of neocortical diffuse plaques—second highest among the first 118 deaths in the Nun Study.

For many older people, concerns about Alzheimer's disease are intensified by the belief that it is inherited and therefore entirely beyond their control. Some genetic vulnerability is almost certainly involved, especially in early-onset Alzheimer's disease (i.e., the form that occurs in middle age). But we know that a purely genetic explanation is almost certainly wrong. Even identical twins who do develop Alzheimer's disease do not do so at the same age, which tells us that nongenetic factors are involved. Nutrition, viral infections, exposure to toxic substances, and other environmental factors yet to be discovered are an important part of the explanation. In Alzheimer's disease, as in so much else about aging, genes are not destiny. How we live also determines how we age.

Most older people fear being confined to a nursing home, and the limitations of such life are undeniable. But only 5 percent of people over the age of sixty-five live in nursing homes, and that percentage has been falling for at least ten years. The rest live in the community at large, and fewer than 5 percent of them need help with the basic activities of daily living.

No doubt the physical performance of older people would be still better if they were more physically active. It is true that the capacity for maximum physical effort declines with age, even in the absence of disease and even among lifelong athletes. Fortunately, demands for such heroic effort are seldom encountered in daily life. Even after a considerable reduction in reserve capacity, older men and women retain a level of physical function that is ample for active living. In chapter 6, we discuss the very optimistic findings about exercise in old age.

The research evidence regarding cognitive (mental) ability in old age, like that for physical ability, is reassuring. There are undeniable age-related declines in cognitive function, but there are three encouraging facts: first, these declines rarely affect all kinds of cognitive performance; second, most of the losses come late in life; and third, many older people are not significantly affected by even minor losses of mental ability.

Functional Loss: Inevitable or Preventable?

Some losses in physical function and in certain kinds of cognitive capacity are indeed intrinsic to age and therefore inevitable. However, the losses experienced in the course of what we have called "usual aging" are a combination of the inevitable and the preventable, more often the latter. People often blame aging for losses that are in fact caused by lifestyle—overeating and poor nutrition, smoking, excessive use of alcohol, lack of regular exercise, and insufficient mental (cognitive) exertion. The couch-potato syndrome, all too common in spite of public ridicule and good resolutions, has both physical and mental effects.

No experiment has made a direct assessment of the effort required for prevention as compared to that for recovery. Logic and experience, however, tell us that preventing a problem is almost always easier than correcting it. Whoever said "an ounce of prevention is worth a pound of cure" may not have made a formal recipe, but the gist is likely accurate. Anyone who has experienced the effort of weight loss in comparison to maintaining normal weight will require no further persuasion.

Lost Forever or Recoverable?

The notion that abilities, once lost in old age, are lost forever is another of the dismal assumptions proved wrong by MacArthur research. We now know that much of the cognitive loss considered intrinsic to aging itself is actually caused by extrinsic factors—for example, not using or challenging the mind on a regular basis. In chapter 8, we discuss ways in which mental abilities can be preserved or even enhanced as we grow older.

Similar evidence for increasing physical performance in old age is already extensive, and we review it in chapters 6 and 7. Older men and women, even those in nursing homes, show substantial gains in muscle strength and aerobic capacity when they follow programs of progressive training. The psychological by-products of such exercise are also important. For instance, just ten weeks of pumping iron (progressive resistance training of the large muscles) brought relief from symptoms of depression, a common problem among older people.

CONTINUING ENGAGEMENT WITH LIFE

In a letter to his daughter in 1908, Freud captured the precious quality of active life in later years:

> *You have, my poor child, seen death break into the family for the first time . . . an[d] perhaps shuddered at the idea that for none of us can life be made any safer. This is something that all we old people know, which is why life for us has such a special value. We refuse to allow the inevitable end to interfere with our happy activities . . . Your loving father.*

MacArthur research shows clearly that our "happy activities" are essential to successful aging. But this is a relatively novel idea.

Thirty years ago, something called "disengagement theory" was influential among gerontologists. This theory defined the main task of old age as letting go. The argument was that old age was a time at which people were required to give up their jobs, could no longer take part in the more strenuous forms of recreation, and sadly, had to say farewell to many old friends and family members. The final act of relinquishment was letting go of life itself.

Fortunately, this theory is much less influential today. In fact, we stress that continued engagement with life is the third important component of successful aging. Maintaining close relationships with others, and remaining involved in activities that are meaningful and purposeful, are important for well-being throughout the life course. And these activities are no less important in later life than in earlier years.

We do not deny that certain losses become more probable with increasing age—the death of friends and loved ones, the often am-bivalent experience of retirement, the necessity of moving away from a familiar house or neighborhood. But the importance of close relationships with others, and of regular activities that give meaning and excitement to life, continues. The task of successful aging is to discover and rediscover relationships and activities that provide closeness and meaningfulness.

Relating to Others

A popular song of a decade ago described the good luck of "people who need people" and, it might have added, "people who are needed by people." Most of us are in both categories and, in spite of the occasional long-lived hermit, being closely related to others is a matter of life and death. Being part of a social network of friends and family is one of the most dependable predictors of longevity. Men and women, perhaps especially men, who do not have close friends or family are more likely to become ill and less likely to live long lives.

The fact that being connected to others promotes health and

longevity was observed long before it was understood, and much research has tried to learn just what it is about such relationships that is good for us. An important part of the answer, as we will explain more fully in chapter 10, has to do with giving and receiving social support. Supportive behavior takes many forms, but it is useful to think of two broad categories, which have been labeled "socio-emotional" and "instrumental." Socio-emotional support includes expressions of affection, respect, and esteem; they assure a person that he or she is valued. Instrumental support involves acts of direct assistance, such as giving physical help, doing or helping with chores, providing transportation, and giving or lending money.

Older men and women are providers as well as receivers of social support, and much of the support that they receive is provided by people in their own age range—husbands and wives, brothers and sisters. Ideally, we can think of each person as moving through life surrounded by others who form a convoy of social support. The size of that convoy, the quality of the relationships within it, and the adequacy of the support it provides are powerful determinants of each person's well-being and quality of life. In chapter 10, we will explore the specific ways in which supportive relationships with others are important for successful aging.

Continuing Productive Activity

Most people, when they think of being productive, think about earning money. Older men and women who run households, care for family members and friends, or volunteer in churches and civic organizations often describe their occupations as "nothing," or "just a housewife," or "I'm retired." These self-deprecating responses underestimate the value of what older people really do, and the importance of their contributions to society.

Our approach to successful aging corrects this bias; we count as productive all activities, paid or unpaid, that create goods or services of value. Using this broader definition, we will see in chapter 11 what older men and women really do with their time, what it takes for them to be productive, and what opportunities for productive activity they would like to have. Finally, we will examine the place of productive activity in the larger pattern of successful aging.

SUCCESSFUL AGING OR THE IMITATION OF YOUTH?

Modern society, perhaps especially American society, seems to regard aging as something to be denied or concealed. Women are freed, happily, from the corsets and similar instruments of torture that fashion once decreed. But a massive and inventive cosmetics industry does its best to persuade middle-aged and elderly women—and increasingly, men—that they will lead happier lives if they change their hair color from gray to some improbable shade of blonde or red, camouflage their hair loss, and cover, erase, or abrade their wrinkles.

Photographs that advertise the products in question show people who are invariably young in appearance; photographer and makeup artist collaborate to send the incessant message of youth. And what cosmetics and computer-enhanced photography cannot do, plastic surgery offers to accomplish. The implication of all this information and misinformation is that the ultimate form of successful aging would be no aging at all. A psychologist might be tempted to say that underlying this denial of the aging process is a more deep-seated denial: refusal to acknowledge the fact of human mortality and the inevitability of death.

Our view of successful aging is not built on the search for immortality and the fountain of youth. George Bernard Shaw, when he was in his nineties, was asked whether he had any advice for younger people. He did. "Do not try to live forever," said Shaw, "you will not succeed." Or, as psychologist Carol Ryff put it in a thoughtful article, "Ponce de León missed the point."

In short, successful aging means just what it says—aging well, which is very different from not aging at all. The three main components of successful aging—avoiding disease and disability, maintaining mental and physical function, and continuing engagement with life—are important throughout life, but their realization in old age differs from that at earlier life stages. We discuss those differences very briefly in this chapter; they are considered more fully in the chapters on each component of successful aging (chapters 5–11).

Avoiding Disease and Disability

Minimizing the risk of disease and disability is of lifelong importance, but some of the risks change with age and, therefore, so do the means for reducing them. For example, the time required to recover from infections and injuries increases markedly with age, as does the possibility that either can cause death. Prevention and avoidance thus become increasingly important. The incidence of specific diseases also changes with age, and the presence of certain chronic diseases becomes more likely. Hypertension and diabetes are examples. Prevention requires increasing attention, therefore, to the symptoms and test results that precede the onset of the diseases themselves.

Even risks that are common to people of all ages may, on analysis, show age-related differences that have implications for successful prevention. For example, auto accidents are a hazard irrespective of age. When the frequency of accidents is analyzed in relation to age and to number of miles driven, young men and older drivers of both sexes appear to be at relatively high risk. The nature of their accidents, however, is very different and so are the means of prevention. For young men, the problem is speed. For older drivers, the prototypical accident involves making a left turn against oncoming traffic, a common maneuver that requires good vision, the ability to estimate the speed of approaching cars, and quick reaction time. Preventive driving for elderly people, therefore, should involve special

caution when making such turns or, better still, avoiding them altogether by making a succession of right turns or by turning left only
where there are left-turn traffic signals.

Maintaining Mental and Physical Function

Gradual decreases in physical reserve and maximum performance are not only age-related; they are to some extent age-
determined. Some adaptation to that fact is therefore necessary. The
eager downhill skier may convert to cross-country skiing, and at an
increasingly sedate pace; the enthusiastic runner may become an
equally enthusiastic jogger or walker. The good news is that moderate regular exercise has many of the benefits of more strenuous ath-
letics. The bad news, all too familiar, is that most older men and
women do not engage even in moderate exercise on a regular basis.
People watch the television commercials that extol the advantages of
exercise, and they buy the machines that promise to flatten their
"abs" and bulge their biceps. But watching and buying provide exercise only to the eyes and the pocketbook, not the body. To maintain
physical function, the body requires more. The forms of appropriate
exercise change with age, as does the intensity of exercise, but the
need for it and the benefits it confers continue throughout life.

The maintenance of cognitive function depends in part on
physical well-being. Exercise, as we shall see in chapter 8, has mental
as well as physical benefits. Beyond that, maintenance of cognitive
ability requires the continued use of the mind, continued engagement in complex cognitive activity. We know that people who perform jobs that require little thought and allow little independent
judgment tend to lose intellectual flexibility, and also reduce the
intellectual content of their leisure activities. People whose jobs are
more interesting, more varied, and demand more problem-solving
skills do not show such job-related losses in mental function.

The special problem for older men and women, most of whom
are retired from employment, is that their retirement has deprived
them of a major source of social and mental stimulation. The solu-

tion, of course, is for them to discover alternative sources of that stimulation, alternative ways of using their cognitive abilities. In chapters 8 and 11, we explore the opportunities for such activities.

Continuing Engagement with Life

Engagement with life, as we have seen, takes two main forms: maintaining relationships with other people, and performing activities that are, in the broadest sense, productive. For much of adult life, employment provides both, although often imperfectly. The fact of earning money is evidence of productivity, and for many people the job gives a more direct sense of meaningful productive contribution. Employment is also, almost always, a social activity; there are co-workers, some of whom become friends. Older people, after retiring from employment, must find appropriate substitute activities and must either find ways to maintain friendships that grew out of work, or replace them.

Society does not make these transitions easy. Old age has been called a "roleless role," a time when it is no longer clear what is expected of the elderly person, or where he or she can find the resources that will make old age successful.

For earlier life stages, the expectations are clearer. Children are expected to attend school; in fact, they are legally required to do so. Able-bodied adults are expected to be employed or to be actively seeking paid employment. Parents of young children are expected to care for them. None of these societal expectations generates perfect compliance, but all of them are felt and most of them are backed by law.

The years after child-rearing and employment present a sharp contrast to these expectational patterns and arrangements for their fulfillment. Almost nothing is expected of the elderly. The spoken advice from youth to age is "take it easy," which means do nothing, or amuse yourself. The unspoken message is "find your own way and keep out of ours."

Many older men and women do better than that. As we shall

see, they find new friends, partially replace paid employment with useful voluntary activity, maintain some form of regular exercise, and enjoy a measure of increased leisure. But many others do much less and age less well. Our purpose is to make the resources for successful aging more widely available, make the content of successful aging more widely understood, and thus increase the numbers of those who age successfully.

SUCCESSFUL AGING: THE RESEARCH PEDIGREE

Successful aging, as we said when we first used the phrase, is an attractive idea. Agreement on its desirability comes easily; agreement on its definition is harder to come by. The lack of agreement about the requirements of successful aging is not for lack of effort. References on the subject go back more than fifty years. Criticisms of those efforts, however, began almost as early, and are at least as numerous. The definitions failed in four respects: 1) they tended to define successful aging in a narrow fashion, favoring one researcher's ideas rather than making a coherent theory of human development; 2) they treated success as no more than the absence of explicit failure, like treating health as nothing more than the absence of explicit disease; 3) they neglected the positive aspects of aging, and possible gains in old age, as if successful aging were merely aging as little as possible; and 4) they failed to acknowledge the unavoidable place of values in defining what is good or bad, successful or unsuccessful.

We have tried to avoid these shortcomings by proposing a research-based model of successful aging, by going beyond absence of disease and disability, and by describing the ways in which personal relationships and productive behavior change as people move through the life course. The MacArthur Study provides the foundation for such a model, and its findings guide us toward a realistic and viable definition of "success" for all older people.

CHAPTER THREE

"Usual Aging"

Older people are stereotyped into two groups—the diseased and the "normal." This is ironic for several reasons. For one, many people placed in the "normal" group are in fact at high risk of disease, but not quite there yet—they may not have reached some arbitrary diagnostic threshold of disease. And these diagnoses are, indeed, arbitrary in many cases: just recently, a small shift in the definition of diabetes created several million diabetics overnight. By calling people who are on the borderline of disease "normal," we underestimate their vulnerability and fail to take protective action on their behalf. That has to change.

The fact is, modest increases in blood pressure, blood sugar, and body weight, and low bone density, are common among "normal" elderly. We tend to view something "normal" as harmless, carrying no risk, as God intended it to be and not subject to change. But while these risk factors are *age-related* in industrial societies, they are not *age-determined* or universal—nor are they harmless. They promote the risk of disease. And they *all* can be modified. We must stop underestimating the power of lifestyle factors such as diet, exercise, and smoking cessation in reducing risk and improving quality of life. When we recognize the importance of lifestyle tools, and learn how to help people realize their potential benefits, we can finally make the move from a gerontology of inevitable decline to one of sustained success.

"USUAL AGING"

We propose the term "usual aging" to describe the elderly who are functioning well, yet are at substantial risk for disease or disability. This is a large percentage of all older people.

At any age, the portion of individuals who are diseased can be divided into those with and without associated disability. For instance, a person found to have an early cancer showing up as a "spot" on a lung X ray, but who has no symptoms, is diseased but not yet disabled. As people grow older, they are more likely to have disability associated with their disease, partly because of the increase in such debilitating health problems as dementia, osteoporosis, cancer, arthritis, and cardiac disease. Traditionally, doctors have focused on caring for the diseased and disabled. But we feel strongly that those who are considered "normal" should often be treated as well. Their blood pressure should be controlled; their weight brought into a normal range; and so on. Too many in this "normal" group have already experienced risky physiological changes, such as modest increases in systolic blood pressure, abdominal fat, and blood sugar and losses in immune system, lung, kidney, or other functions, all of which set the stage for development of disease. They suffer, often silently, from the syndrome of "usual aging," a condition associated with significant risk of disease and premature death.

RISKS OF "USUAL AGING"

"Usual aging" involves two key sets of problems. First, many body organs, including the kidneys, heart, and lungs, gradually lose strength with advancing age. Immune function also declines with age. These changes place the elderly at risk for disease or dysfunction, especially in the presence of major stress. The second set of problems that develop in "usual aging" relate to the buildup of many risky characteristics such as high levels of blood fats and sugar, hypertension, and so on.

Let's consider the impact of each type of decline associated with "usual aging."

First, take the case of general decline in recuperative power. Imagine a thirty-year-old man and his eighty-year-old grandfather who are exposed to bacteria known to cause lung infection. Both develop pneumonia in the lower lobe of their right lung. The younger man is likely to experience fever, coughing, some chest discomfort, and general weakness. With proper diagnosis and administration of the correct antibiotic, he recovers promptly, perhaps losing only a couple of days or a week from work. His grandfather, on the other hand, with the same pneumonia, in the same lobe of the same lung, is not likely to fare nearly as well. His initial symptoms may be the same. But even if the diagnosis is made at the same time as in his grandson and he is also given the appropriate antibiotic, the course of his illness might be very grave indeed. This is because the average healthy eighty-year-old nonsmoker has only about two-thirds the lung function of his thirty-year-old counterpart—and his immune system is impaired as well. With this perilous double jeopardy, the grandfather's pneumonia may spread to other lung areas. He may require administration of oxygen or even be placed on a ventilator. The infection may spread to his bloodstream and perhaps to other organs. The scene is set for the emergence of a life-threatening illness in this older person. And the difference between young and old is purely related to the physiologic consequences of "usual aging."

A second example of the general health decline in old age can be seen in the dramatic age-related increase in the likelihood of mortality from third-degree burns. For instance, a burn covering 35 percent of the body surface would kill half the victims aged thirty-five to forty-nine, while a burn covering just 15 percent of the body would kill the same percentage of victims aged sixty to seventy-four years. By age seventy-five and over, a burn covering just 10 percent of the body would kill half of the victims, and so on. The older the person, the less extensive the burn needs to be to kill half the victims. This reflects the multiple, simultaneous, age-related reductions throughout middle and old age in lung, kidney, immune system, and cardiac function—all of which are called upon to respond to the overwhelming stress of a major burn. That this effect is evident in late midlife, well before many diseases become prevalent, shows the impact of "usual aging," rather than disease.

Now let's look beyond the gradual age-related losses of function to the second type of increased risk associated with "usual aging"— that is, the often subtle, common, risky abnormalities that emerge in many people in middle and late life. These include modest increases in blood sugar and insulin, body fat (especially in the abdomen where it is more risky), and blood pressure, and a general reduction in immune functions. These "usual aging" characteristics increase the risk of important diseases in late life. And yet they are often considered "normal" by many health care providers. It is not unusual for a physician to indicate to an older person that her systolic blood pressure and blood sugar might be a little high, but they are "okay for your age, my dear." This statement, while meant to encourage rather than alarm the patient, implies that the criteria for normal health are age-related, and that her increases in blood pressure and blood sugar carry no risks. Nothing could be farther from the truth.

Consider the risks of high blood sugar and high insulin levels, known as the "pseudodiabetes" of aging. This is a common, and worrisome, feature of the "usual aging" syndrome. Pseudodiabetes of aging carries substantial risk of adverse health problems, whether or not the person actually develops full-blown diabetes. Both high sugar and insulin levels increase the risk of coronary heart disease. Increasing levels of blood sugar within the previously considered "normal" range carry very substantial risk. The higher the level of blood sugar, the greater the risk of both stroke and heart attack.

Variability

Just as no two people are alike, so their physiological health—that is, the functional capacity of their major body organs—varies dramatically. This variability between individuals tends to increase substantially with advancing age. Thus it is fair to say that the older people become, the more dissimilar they become. If you have seen one old person, you have not seen them all. We must fight the tendency to overgeneralize about the health and abilities of older people.

Reversing Usual Aging

We have established the fact that a great portion of "usual aging" risks can be modified with positive shifts in lifestyle. Now, let's look briefly at the kinds of changes that make a meaningful difference. A recent study of "usual aging" looked at middle-aged and older men at risk of heart disease. The study compared the effects of a nine-month diet-induced weight loss (approximately 10 percent of body weight) to the effects of a constant-weight aerobic exercise program. The study participants were initially obese, had modest increases in blood pressure, blood sugar, insulin, and a blood fat profile conducive to the development of vascular disease. In short, they were quite typical of the "usual aging" syndrome of multiple risk factors for major diseases.

The low-calorie diet caused significant reductions in weight, blood sugar, insulin levels, blood pressure, and blood levels of cholesterol and triglycerides. The "good cholesterol," or HDL, increased. In sum, the diet improved or reversed every single risk factor. While the older weight loss subjects (over sixty years) lost less weight than the middle-aged subjects and had more modest improvements in blood sugar levels, they participated fully in the reductions of all other risk factors. In general, the weight loss intervention had greater effects than the constant-weight aerobic exercise program.

The Benefits of Treating "Usual Aging"

It is one thing to demonstrate the modifiability of "usual aging" risk factors, but to provide clinically useful advice, we must also show a bottom line effect—that is, demonstrate that changes in lifestyle actually decrease the risk of disease or death. It's not enough just to lower blood sugar or blood pressure. The critical question is, does that translate into better overall health and/or longer life? Happily, we do now have those answers. One important study of systolic hypertension showed that after an average of 4.5 years of standard treatment which effectively lowered blood pressure (with very few side effects), the incidence of stroke was 36 percent lower, and the incidence of heart attacks was 27 percent lower, in the treatment group. Even those over eighty years old saw the health benefits of blood pressure reduction, regardless of race or gender. These results strengthen our belief that the risk factors that comprise the "usual aging" syndrome are modifiable. But even more important, they highlight the value of identifying people at risk, and targeting aggressive prevention strategies to this segment of the older population. To a much greater degree than previously recognized, we are responsible for our own health status in old age.

CHAPTER FOUR

NATURE VERSUS NURTURE
IN AGING

T HE RELATIVE IMPORTANCE of nature (inheritance) and nurture (environment) to issues as wide-ranging as schizophrenia, breast cancer, and homosexuality has recently captured the interest of scientists and the general public. The dramatic discoveries of genetic research emphasize the importance of heredity, and popular wisdom dictates that the secret to a long, healthful life lies in choosing your parents wisely. Most people seem to feel that how well one ages is hereditary, and when asked how they expect to age, many refer to their parent's pattern of aging or the ages at which their parents or siblings died. Comments such as "I come from long-lived stock" or "no male in my family has lived past sixty-five" are common. But while most people assume that genes play the dominant role, new research suggests that environment and lifestyle may in fact be more important in terms of the risk factors associated with aging. This holds true for many of the most common risk factors for heart disease, as an example. And since environmental effects are more likely than genetic ones to be changeable, the fact that the environment is a powerful influence on aging suggests a very optimistic scenario. For if we can avoid, or modify, many of the risk factors that affect the aging process, we can better control our health destiny.

Furthermore, genetic influence does not necessarily mean that a risk factor cannot be modified. Nature and nurture interact, and in many cases, the effects of the genes can be avoided or modified by appropriate lifestyle changes and medical treatments.

We use a tool called the *heritability index* to determine the proportion of a disease, personality trait, or physical characteristic attributable to genetic influences. It's a very useful measure, and one that can be used to determine the relative importance of genetics and environment at different ages. For instance, a given characteristic might be largely determined by one's genes at age forty, but the same characteristic might be determined more powerfully by lifestyle at age eighty. Why should this matter to you? Because once you know how much your genes dictate, and how much your environment and habits control, you can seize the opportunity to make lifesaving changes in your behavior—at any age.

Distinguishing Nature from Nurture

How do we learn the relative importance of nature and nurture? There are several ways, and we describe them here in order to show you just how persuasive the MacArthur data really are.

The simplest method involves family studies in which patterns of disease, personality traits, or physical characteristics are measured in family members of two or more generations. This is particularly effective when a disorder or characteristic is determined by a single identifiable gene, as it is for some forms of breast cancer or early-onset Alzheimer's disease. The usefulness of such family studies is limited, however, since family members are reared in the same household and often share many aspects of their environment—including similar diets, child-rearing patterns, education, and the like.

A second strategy is to study populations that have changed their environment. For instance, studies have found that stomach cancer is less common in Japanese living in the United States than for those living in Japan, suggesting that diet, or another environmental factor, plays a major role in the development of stomach cancer. But it's hard to prove specific cause and effect in such studies.

A third strategy is adoption studies, in which individuals adopted early in life are compared to their adoptive (nonbiological) family members as well as to their biological parents and siblings. When applied to studies of obesity, as discussed in detail later, such studies indicate that fatness is predominantly inherited, since adopted individuals resemble their biological parents more than they resemble their adoptive parents. But this strategy is limited by the fact that proper identification of both biologic parents can be difficult—causing uncertainty about genetic forces.

A final method, the study of twins, was used in the MacArthur Study. Twin studies are an exceptional tool for dissecting nature from nurture. Identical twins share identical genetic complements, while nonidentical twins share, on average, 50 percent of their genes. The MacArthur studies used one of the largest and most widely studied of registries, the Swedish National Twin Registry, which includes a total of nearly 25,000 sets of same-sex twins born in Sweden between 1886 and 1958. This information has recently been extensively analyzed in the MacArthur Studies of Successful Aging and has yielded fascinating results. The information is even more substantial because some of the twins in the registry were separated at birth, which removes the potential confusion of nature and nurture. MacArthur researchers were thus able to get a solid grip on the relative importance of genes and environment in aging. Here's what they found.

Obesity

Genes account for slightly more than two-thirds of the risk for obesity—which should come as welcome news to older overweight individuals who have long contended that "it's in my genes!" But it also shows that one has to work against a significant obstacle—

heredity—to be of normal weight. Does this mean that it's okay to throw in the towel and eat Twinkies all day long, saying, "It's not my fault!"? Far from it. This still leaves room for the influence of diet, exercise, and other factors. Even genetically preprogrammed risk factors can be modified with good old-fashioned willpower.

Blood Pressure

Blood pressure rises with advancing age, especially systolic pressure (the higher of the two numbers routinely reported for blood pressure). Recent research shows that the modest increases in systolic pressure which occur in nearly half of the elderly are an important risk factor for the development of stroke. The riskiness of isolated systolic hypertension, a common condition in older people, and the value of its treatment are discussed more fully in chapter 5. Research has found that when it comes to the risk of high blood pressure, lifestyle factors are increasingly important—and genes less important—with advancing age.

Blood Fat Levels (Cholesterol) and Triglycerides

It is well known that high blood levels of the lipids (fats) cholesterol and triglycerides, for example, influence the risk of developing coronary heart disease, the number-one cause of death in the United States, in middle age. Prevention efforts have focused on lowering blood fats with exercise, diet, and medication. Most people seem to assume that cholesterol levels are partly the result of intrinsic factors (one's "metabolism") and partly the result of diet. The MacArthur Study now offers firm evidence as to the role of nature and nurture in determining cholesterol and other blood fat levels. The study found a substantial genetic influence for both cholesterol and triglycerides. But it also showed that genes become much less important as one ages. In fact, when it comes to high triglyceride levels—a strong risk factor for repeat heart attacks—genes play no role whatsoever among people over seventy. That's right—triglyceride levels are entirely determined by lifestyle in this older population, and that means one can effectively decide if one wants to lower those levels or not by eating fewer sugary foods, lowering alcohol intake, exercising more, and other healthy lifestyle measures. Triglycerides are thus an extreme example of the general finding that the older one becomes, the less important heredity becomes—and the more dominant becomes one's lifestyle.

Lung Function

Not only is lung disease common among the elderly, but even in those without evidence of lung disease, the lungs become stiffer, weaker, and less effective with age. A strong association is found between low lung function and future development of coronary heart disease, whether or not one smokes or has chronic obstructive pulmonary disease or lung cancer. The total amount of air inhaled in one's deepest breath and the fastest rate at which one can exhale are powerful predictors of how many more years one will live. These measures of lung function have been proposed as "biomarkers" of age and may reflect broad aspects of total body aging. What is the relative importance of genes and environment in terms of decreasing lung function with age? Just as with hypertension and high cholesterol, the older one gets, the less significant is the role of genes on lung function. Lifestyle habits are the most critical factors, and a sedentary lifestyle is the greatest risk factor in this case.

Mental Sharpness

A recent major study of twins over eighty years of age looked at the impact on genes on mental functioning. The overall findings were as follows: when you look at general mental ability, verbal skills, spatial skills, thinking speed, and memory, you find that about half of all mental loss with age can be attributed to genes. The other half is related to lifestyle and environment. In other words, there's a lot one can do to keep one's mind sharp with age. Just as we must keep our physical selves active, so we must keep our minds busy in our later years if we want it to continue to function well. We discuss this in greater detail in chapter 8. "Use it or lose it" is a mental, not just a physical, phenomenon.

Pseudodiabetes of Aging

When we look at the so-called pseudodiabetes of aging, a common condition in which blood sugar and insulin levels rise, a similar pattern emerges. While genes are important, external factors may play a stronger role. For instance, factors that impair sugar metabolism include increases in the percentage of body fat (especially potbelly), lack of exercise, poor nutrition, and many medications. Several studies have evaluated the contributions of these external factors to the modifications in sugar metabolism so often associated with aging. A great deal of research has shown that such factors as diet, exercise, and medication are more important than age and genes in determining the risk of pseudodiabetes. Older individuals who are physically fit have substantially better sugar metabolism than their less fit counterparts. Thus, a growing body of evidence suggests that the pseudodiabetes seen in older people, which has long been considered an age-dependent process, may be, in large part, related to other factors, not the biology of aging.

We've been talking about the fact that genes play an increasingly minor role in promotion of *single* risk factors, such as hypertension and high blood fats, with advancing age. But even more important, the same can be said for the risk of full-blown disease, such as coronary heart disease. The older one gets, the less important genes become—and the more important become lifestyle and environment—in promoting this life-threatening risk.

Interaction of Nature and Nurture

While genetic factors are not the dominant causes of risk factors in aging, they do play an important role. But contrary to popular

belief, there is much we can do to decrease our genetically determined risk, since environment often determines the ultimate impact
of genes. By harnessing the power of proper diet, exercise, smoking
cessation, and so on, we can prevent or defuse a potential genetic
time bomb.

CHAPTER FIVE

AVOIDING DISEASE AND DISABILITY IN LATE LIFE

MACARTHUR RESEARCH SHOWS us again and again that we need not hope for just added years—we can, and should, strive for longer, healthier, more productive lives. The notion that we can attain high-quality, vital, disease-free late years is a novel one. Even recently, it would have seemed paradoxical to discuss health promotion and disease prevention in the elderly. Most prevention studies excluded elderly subjects. This form of ageism was based on the prevalent myth that "the horse is out of the barn," and reflected the widespread feelings of older people and health care providers that it's impossible to change habits that have been ingrained over decades, and that even if you could change your lifestyle, it is unlikely your aged body would respond to improve function and reduce risk. For instance, when encouraged to quit smoking, an elderly man might respond, "I've had a million of these cigarettes, Doc, no use in my quitting now. Talk to my grandson."

These attitudes stand in contrast to the increasing evidence of the remarkable capacity of older individuals to recover lost function. Time and again it has been shown that physiological conditions of older individuals can be improved to the point of reducing risk. For example, the risk of heart disease falls when you quit smoking regardless of your age, the length of time you have smoked, or how heavy a smoker you are. True, this can mean added pressure on older people to take stock and take action. But there is a prize—and it may mean sitting on a bike instead of in a wheelchair at age ninety.

With the remarkable increases in longevity, and increasing awareness that risks associated with advancing age may be reversible, health *promotion,* not just disease prevention, is emerging as an important theme in geriatrics. The goal of these efforts in old age need not always be prevention—sometimes delay is really all we need. The benefits of delaying the onset of disease are very substantial, and problems in old age such as heart disease and cancer are often subject to delay, if not to prevention. Since many individuals in their eighth and ninth decades of life have many life-threatening conditions at once, delay in the emergence of a single disease, such as cancer, for as much as five years will dramatically reduce disability, suffering, and the cost of medical care. This reduction in the total period of disability—formally known as "compression of morbidity"—is the main goal of prevention initiatives in late life. The nice thing is, however, that some of the same lifestyle changes that reduce the risk of one disease may delay, or cut the risk of, others as well.

Let's take a look at the potential to delay major diseases and thereby prolong life. Mortality from heart disease declined more than 50 percent between 1958 and 1992. In the famous Framingham Heart Study, if older individuals had been able to reduce their risk factors for heart disease, the men would have survived to 100 years of age and the women to ninety-seven years of age. And remember this: they would potentially have lived both longer *and* healthier lives.

A major concern regarding changing risk in older persons is the *latency* of the effects of health promotion initiatives. Many individuals feel that it takes a long time for any change in health habits to reduce the risk of a disease, and thus it is not worthwhile to implement such initiatives late in life. What's the point, they ask, of working hard to promote health benefits a person won't likely live to see? However, research has clearly shown that interventions such as smoking cessation in older people reduces risk as promptly (within months) as in younger individuals.

While this information suggests that older people should take part in health promotion and disease prevention initiatives, some caveats exist before we rush headlong into this area. We should not blindly generalize the findings of studies in middle age or younger individuals to the elderly just because the disease that we are attempting to prevent, for instance, heart attack, occurs in old people as well as their middle-aged counterparts. The organs of older persons differ significantly from younger adults and we should not assume that what works for middle-aged people also works for older ones. For instance, while it has been well documented that high total serum cholesterol levels increase the risk for developing heart disease in middle age, this is still a controversial issue in older people. And as we will discuss in more detail later in this chapter, there is good reason to doubt whether strict dietary or medication attempts to reduce cholesterol levels are beneficial in old age. On the positive side, however, there are many ways in which lifestyle changes have been clearly proved to benefit the elderly. Here are some of those ways.

PREVENTION OF SPECIFIC DISEASES IN OLD AGE

Exercise and Physical Activity as Prevention Strategies

MacArthur research shows that exercise can benefit the older population tremendously. It helps prevent heart disease, high blood pressure, and the tendency toward diabetes. In addition, important information is now available on the role of physical activity in decreasing the risk of problems as diverse as some cancers, osteoporosis, and falls in older people. Given its very substantial importance and the rapidly enlarging body of scientific information currently available, exercise in old age is discussed in detail in chapter 6 of this book. Accordingly, in the recommendations regarding prevention of heart disease, stroke, and specific cancers presented in this chapter, we touch on the role of exercise in less detail.

PREVENTION AND EARLY DETECTION OF CANCER IN OLD AGE

The increase with advancing age in the incidence of most cancers is due to several factors. First, a buildup of "errors" in cells has been implicated in the development of age-related cancers, including prostate, multiple myeloma, and chronic lymphocytic leukemia. Second, the delayed effect of factors such as exposure to environmental carcinogens starts to appear in later life. For instance, mesothelioma—a highly malignant tumor of the lung lining—occurs decades after exposure to the inciting agent, asbestos. Third, the *cumulative* effect of environmental or lifestyle-related risk factors such as sun exposure (skin cancer), certain dietary factors (colon cancer), or smoking (lung and other cancers) comes into play as we age. The longer one lives, the greater the cumulative impact of these risk factors, and the greater the risk of developing cancer.

Aside from its effect on survival, cancer is often a chronic disease that robs life from years, causing substantial pain, suffering, and loss of function as well as increasing health care costs. As efforts to reduce death rates from heart attack and stroke cut these death rates in older people, cancer is likely to emerge as the major cause of death and disability in old age. But some types of cancer can be prevented, and it's never too late to start trying. While cancer prevention has focused on middle age and the old are often excluded from studies of cancer risk, substantial information has recently emerged to guide cancer prevention efforts in late life.

There are two key ways to avoid serious problems associated with cancer. One is to prevent it in the first place (a preferable choice); the other is to catch it early, when the chance of a cure is greatest. Early detection is becoming increasingly important today, since most forms of cancer are treatable and the treatments are most effective, least costly, and associated with least complications in the early stage of the disease. Our recommendations here are drawn from major, recognized cancer organizations. However, where there is controversy or specific relevant research is lacking, we on occasion offer our own professional opinions.

BREAST CANCER

Detection: Breast cancer, common in older women, responds well to treatments such as surgery, radiation, and chemotherapy. It also often grows more slowly in older women than in premenopausal women. All women, regardless of age, should learn the proper techniques of monthly breast self-examination. In addition, it is important to have an annual breast examination by a physician or a trained nurse practitioner.

Mammography (X-ray examination of the breast) is a sensitive and effective tool for early detection of breast cancer, and should be performed routinely on older women as well as younger ones. Most leading authorities now agree that women should have mammograms every year from age forty to age eighty. Women known to be at high risk, including those with prior breast cancer or other breast disease, or a family history of breast cancer in their mother or sisters, may require more frequent screening at their doctors' discretion. However, it should be noted that about three-quarters of women who develop breast cancer have no family history of the disease. So screening is important for *all* women. Medicare now covers annual mammograms for all women aged forty and over and waives the deductible for the procedure.

Prevention: There are several things one may be able to do to lessen the chance of developing breast cancer. Hormone replacement therapy for postmenopausal women, while it has many health benefits, does increase the risk of breast cancer by 30 to 50 percent, regardless of whether the hormone treatment is estrogen alone or estrogen in combination with progestin. (Many women take the combination hormone regimen, since estrogen alone may promote uterine cancer and added progestins blunt that risk.) The longer one takes hormone replacement, the greater the risk of breast cancer. Just how great is the increased risk? Though 30 to 50 percent may sound like a large amount, for postmenopausal women it boosts the likelihood of developing breast cancer in the next decade from 3 to 4 percent without estrogen to about 5 percent with estrogens—quite a small increase. Clearly this risk is not meaningless, but it must be weighed against the many strong benefits of estrogen replacement after menopause. (We discuss these benefits further on pages 80, 89, and 93.)

For unknown reasons (perhaps related to the tendency of estrogen levels to increase body fat), obesity is also associated with modest increases in the risk of breast cancer. While there has been much discussion and some useful research on the role of nutrition in breast cancer, the findings thus far are meager and certainly not sufficient to recommend specific dietary intakes or avoidance of specific foods. One major study found that women who eat the largest quantities of fruits and vegetables have a lower risk of breast cancer. While this requires further study, there is certainly no harm—and lots to be gained—from eating five to nine servings of fruits and vegetables per day, as recommended by the National Cancer Institute. You may have also heard that excessive alcohol intake is associated with a higher risk of breast cancer. While this may be true, there is far too little data to give women specific advice on how little—if any—alcohol to consume to cut the risk of breast cancer. And finally, despite numerous studies, there is no strong data regarding any association between physical activity and the development of breast cancer.

CERVICAL CANCER

Detection: One of the biggest success stories in the war against cancer has been in the fight against cancer of the cervix. Pelvic examination and PAP smears of the cervix are highly effective tools for early detection of cervical cancer. In fact, many believe that the vast majority of women who die of this cancer failed to be screened. Regardless of her age, a woman who has never had a PAP smear should have annual smears until she has had at least two, and preferably three, negative tests at least one year apart. Most women enter late life having had regular PAP smears. Women over sixty-five years of age do not require regular PAP smears if they have had at least three prior normal smears. They should confer with their doctors about the ideal screening regimen for them. As with all forms of cancer, women of any age who are at increased risk (which for cervical cancer includes a history of prior cervical disease, any sexually transmitted disease or multiple sex partners, and cigarette smoking) should have annual screening. Medicare covers pelvic exam and PAP smear every three years for women at average risk. Annual screening is covered for women at high risk of cervical cancer.

COLON AND RECTAL CANCER

Detection: For colon and rectal cancer, as with many cancers, the absence of proven preventive measures means that the secret to survival lies in early detection. The good news, again, is that screening tests do work in this case. All older people should have an annual rectal examination by a health provider, plus testing of a stool sample for evidence of occult (hidden) bleeding. In addition, at three- to five-year intervals, all older people should have an examination of the rectum and lower colon using an instrument called a flexible sigmoidoscope. This examination can be conducted by an internist or family physician (a specialist is not required). It is not very uncomfortable or expensive, and is *very* effective in detecting early cancer. Medicare now covers colorectal cancer screening tests, including flexible sigmoidoscopy for people aged fifty and over (once every four years), and one screening colonoscopy for high-risk individuals every two years.

Prevention: Eating excessive fat, especially saturated fats, and protein (especially in meat or dairy products) has been implicated as a risk factor for the development of colorectal cancer. Conversely, diets high in fiber, especially cellulose and wheat bran, may protect against colon and rectal cancers. These types of fiber are found in whole grain breads, cereals, and fruits. While the jury is still out on any protective effect of dietary supplements such as vitamins C and E and beta-carotene, most of the available evidence finds them to be of no or very limited value in decreasing colon cancer risk. On the other hand, while definitive evidence is not yet available, the bulk of present knowledge shows that daily aspirin use does protect against colorectal cancers. As with many forms of cancer, cigarette smoking increases the risk of these cancers as well.

Regular exercise may play an important role in the prevention of colon cancer, but not rectal cancer.

PROSTATE CANCER

Detection: Prostate cancer is the most common cancer among American men, and it can be hard to detect. The annual rectal examination, which is an essential screening tool for colon and rectal cancer, is also recommended for all older men for detection of prostate cancer. Several years ago a new blood test, called the PSA test (for Prostate Specific Antigen), became available. High PSA levels in the blood are seen in the presence of prostate cancer, but can also be seen in cases of marked enlargement of the prostate (Benign Prostatic Hyperplasia, which is very common in older men). PSA also appears in the blood with inflammation of a noncancerous prostate gland. For this reason, there is some controversy over the use of the PSA test to screen for prostate cancer. Significant increases in serial measurements of PSA, at six-month or annual intervals, *do* suggest growing prostate cancer.

Some experts still raise controversy over the value of PSA screening for men with normal rectal exams. While the generally accepted upper limit of normal for PSA is 4.0 ng/ml, more than 20 percent of men found to have prostate cancer have PSA levels below this limit. For men with modestly elevated PSA levels, say, in the 2.6 to 4.0 range, a new test, called the "Free PSA" test, may be useful. This test could reduce the number of people subjected to invasive prostate biopsies, which are tests of cells in the prostate to see if they're cancerous. If the PSA is lower than 2.0, as is the case for almost three-quarters of men between the ages of fifty and seventy, the risk of cancer is low—and regular PSA screening is probably safe at two-year intervals. The American Cancer Society and the American Urological Society recommend annual PSA determinations, in conjunction with rectal exam, for men aged fifty to seventy years. But the American College of Physicians and the United States Preventive Service Task Force have not endorsed routine screening. Medicare now covers an annual prostate cancer screening test for men aged fifty and over. This test may include either or both of the following: a digital rectal exam and a prostate-specific antigen blood test.

Many older men with high PSA levels who are found on further testing to have cancer isolated to the prostate gland are gripped by the psychological stress of the diagnosis, then exposed to aggressive surgical treatment, such as radical prostatectomy, which may result in complications such as impotence or incontinence. For men found to have modestly elevated PSA levels, the "Free PSA" measurement may be useful in determining if the PSA level is truly of concern.

Prevention: The risk of prostate cancer is higher in countries in which diet is rich in animal fat and proteins. But this information is not yet well enough developed to permit specific recommendations or even warnings. Similarly, while there has been much discussion on the possible relationship between physical activity and the development of prostate cancer, the studies to date are inconclusive. One of the many cautions regarding administration of testosterone to older impotent men is the concern that the treatment might hasten the growth of previously undetected prostate cancer.

LUNG CANCER

Detection: Would that there was an effective screening test for lung cancer, one of the leading killers of men and women. As smoking is the major risk factor for lung cancer, several studies have been undertaken to routinely screen smokers with chest X rays or examination of their sputum for cancer cells in an effort toward early detection. Unfortunately, none of these efforts is effective in enhancing survival, and there is now consensus among leading experts that such routine X-ray or sputum screening is not valuable and is not recommended.

Prevention: Smoking causes lung cancer. The more you smoke, the greater your risk, at any age. Filtered cigarettes may be slightly less risky than nonfilters. Pipe and cigar smokers are also at risk. While their risk of lung cancer is lower than that of cigarette smokers, they carry the same risk as cigarette smokers for oral cancer. If you quit smoking, your risk of lung cancer falls as your lungs "heal" the damage caused by the smoking. By the time you have quit for fifteen years, your risk of lung cancer is almost as low as if you had never smoked. Recent attempts to decrease the risk of lung cancer in smokers by taking vitamin E or beta-carotene dietary supplements have not proven successful, but there is some suggestion that daily dietary supplements of selenium (200 mg per day) may decrease the risk. The answer is not to take vitamins, but to quit smoking now!

SKIN CANCER

Detection: Skin cancer is common, and in most cases, easily detected and treated. Certain forms, however, such as melanoma, can be very troublesome and even fatal if not detected and treated early. Thorough skin examination should be part of a regular medical examination for older persons, and rapidly changing or bleeding skin lesions should be promptly brought to the attention of a physician.

Prevention: With advancing age, skin pigment declines, increasing the penetration of sunlight and ultraviolet A-related damage. This promotes the development of precancerous and cancerous growths. The advent of sunscreens has markedly enhanced the ability to prevent skin cancer, while still permitting participation in outdoor activities. To avoid sun damage, sunscreens of at least SPF (Sun Protective Factor) 15 should be used—preferably applied twenty minutes to two hours before sun exposure, and reapplied after swimming or strenuous exercise that may lead to dilution of the sunscreen from water or perspiration. Be sure to use enough sunscreen to cover your entire body, particularly those areas that are easy to forget—the ears, lips, back of the neck, and so on. In addition to sunscreens, the age-old advice of staying out of the midday sun and wearing protective clothing bears repeating.

PREVENTION OF HEART DISEASE AND STROKE

Since coronary artery (heart) disease and stroke are both often reflections of general vascular disease, they tend to have many risk factors in common, such as smoking and high blood pressure. For this reason, the two disorders also share many prevention strategies. Thus there is considerable overlap in our discussion of how to prevent heart disease and stroke.

The advice regarding prevention of coronary artery disease and stroke provided here is intended as a guide for older persons who are healthy and do not have evidence of disease. Guidelines regarding avoidance of a *second* heart attack or stroke, or the aggravation of previously detected evidence of heart disease, may differ. People at high risk should consult their physicians for advice tailored to their specific needs. For instance, people with chronic or intermittent atrial fibrillation, a disturbance of heart rhythm quite common in older people, require chronic treatment with blood thinners, such as coumadin, and close monitoring by a physician in order to lower the risk of stroke.

HEART DISEASE

Heart disease is a major killer of men at all ages, and of older women. After age sixty, heart disease is the primary cause of death in both men and women, killing one in four. While much of the advice given to middle-aged men and women regarding prevention of heart disease also holds for older people (i.e., don't smoke, be lean, etc.), there are some important differences in risk factors among the elderly.

Cholesterol and Other Blood Lipids

America has become obsessed with cholesterol, and for good reason. Elevations in blood cholesterol level are a major risk factor for the development of coronary heart disease—that form of heart disease that leads to chest pain and heart attacks. In otherwise healthy middle-aged men and probably also in women, reduction in total cholesterol levels, through diet or drug treatment, reduces the risk of developing or dying from coronary heart disease. These facts, and the constant barrage of cholesterol-related information in food advertisements and from pharmaceutical companies, understandably lead the elderly and their physicians to take notice. They have tended to apply the concerns about cholesterol in middle-aged individuals to older people.

Not so fast! Caution is advised here. The good news is, cholesterol is not nearly as important a risk factor for the development of coronary heart disease in old age as in middle age. Most studies either find that an older person's total cholesterol is not a risk factor at all, or is a very minor one. For instance, in one major study, elevated total cholesterol (over 240 mg/dl) was a modest risk factor for older women, but not for men. Interestingly, the protective effect of high levels of HDL cholesterol—the "good cholesterol"—appears to continue into old age.

In general, older persons without known heart disease are probably best off not having their total cholesterol measured. This might be somewhat difficult in today's medical environment. If a total cholesterol level is measured and found to be high in an older person, this should not cause alarm. It is best to relax, calm the family, avoid taking medications that have potentially serious side effects, and proceed with life. If low HDL levels are detected, it is probably worth some efforts to increase this "good cholesterol" with exercise (discussed later). It would also be wise to get other risk factors under control. If a high HDL level is detected in an older person, there is nothing to do but brag about it!

Smoking

The facts on smoking as a risk factor for coronary heart disease are beyond dispute. The more you smoke, the greater your risk, at any age. Those who smoke a pack a day have a risk of coronary heart disease nearly four times that of nonsmokers, and even those who smoke less than half a pack a day have twice the risk of nonsmokers. The good news is that the benefits of quitting smoking are substantial, at any age. Surprisingly, after cessation of smoking, the risk of coronary heart disease falls abruptly within months, and within three to five years the risk of coronary heart disease falls to a level indistinguishable from that of individuals who have never smoked. This reduction in risk after quitting is much quicker than that for the risk of lung cancer. These findings hold regardless of how long you have smoked or how much. If that fails to motivate, what will?

Of special news to the elderly is the fact that smoking is age-blind. While the risks of smoking persist into old age, so do the benefits of smoking cessation. Also, regular physical exercise and maintaining a high level of physical fitness may in fact represent in part an *antidote* for the effects of smoking. This is encouraging, especially for smokers, but more research needs to be done in this area.

Hypertension

Hypertension, an increase in blood pressure, occurs in over 60 percent of older persons and comes in two basic forms. The first form, elevation of only systolic pressure (the higher of the two numbers frequently reported for blood pressure) is termed Isolated Systolic Hypertension (ISH). ISH, generally defined as systolic pressure greater than 160 mmHg (with diastolic pressure at 90 mmHg), occurs with increasing frequency over the age of sixty. Nearly a quarter of all older people have this risky condition. For many years, ISH was considered a manifestation of "normal" aging, due to the stiffening of blood vessels with advancing age. Recently ISH has been recognized as a very important component of usual aging, since it is common, dangerous, and most important, modifiable.

ISH is a well-established risk factor for coronary heart disease and stroke. A major study, the Systolic Hypertension in the Elderly Program (SHEP), has shown unequivocally that ISH can be treated easily with common and inexpensive medications such as diuretics (water reduction pills). Best of all, there were few side effects and very substantial reductions in the risks of heart attack and stroke.

The second form of hypertension, with increases in both the top and bottom blood pressure measurements, is also increasingly common with advancing age. Studies have shown the unequivocal benefit of treating this form of hypertension in older persons, which reduces the risk of both coronary heart disease and congestive heart failure. Aggressive management of hypertension, while valuable in all people, appears to be especially critical in diabetics, who are at increased risk of the development of heart disease. In addition, regular physical activity, to be discussed later, clearly delays the development of high blood pressure, and reduces blood pressure in people who already have hypertension. The bottom line is clear: hypertension is neither harmless nor inevitable in old age. Aggressive treatment can save your life.

Syndrome X—Insulin Resistance and Diabetes Mellitus

Syndrome X is a name given to a collection of risky characteristics, including obesity (especially the "northern or potbellied variety," which is more common in men), a tendency toward diabetes, high blood pressure, and high blood fats. This syndrome was once thought to be normal for older people. But as with ISH, it is now known to be a worrisome part of "usual aging"—common, risky, and modifiable. This treacherous mix of risk factors is closely tied to obesity, which stimulates a cascade leading to the other long list of problems. The end result, for many, is coronary heart disease.

But this domino effect is avoidable. A recent important study has shown that Syndrome X is preventable through diet and exercise. Diet-induced weight loss yields slightly greater benefits than weight loss through aerobic exercise alone. However, it is unquestionable that regular exercise can also significantly reduce the chance of developing Syndrome X in the first place, and can also delay the onset of noninsulin-dependent diabetes (type 2 diabetes). This form of diabetes is especially common in older people, and seems to be an advanced form of Syndrome X in some people. Tackling or preventing Syndrome X in older people promises to be a dramatic advance in health promotion and disease prevention efforts in this population.

Postmenopausal Hormone Replacement Therapy

The dramatic increase in heart disease in women after menopause has led to the belief that replacement with estrogen, and more recently cyclic estrogen-progestin combinations, will convey some protection. Numerous studies have investigated this issue, most notably the Nurses Health Study, a very large prospective study which has now reported data on this question for over 59,000 women followed for sixteen years. The consensus of this research is that postmenopausal hormone replacement reduces the risk of heart disease an average of 44 percent, and increases life expectancy by three years—a dramatic effect. Today, most postmenopausal women who have not had a hysterectomy choose estrogen-progestin combinations, which probably carry less risk than estrogen alone. Women who take cyclic estrogen-progestin combinations have a 61 percent lower risk of developing heart disease than women who take no postmenopausal hormone replacement. While the difference between estrogen alone (44 percent) and estrogen-progestin (61 percent) in protecting against heart disease may not be statistically significant, the balance of the available data indicates that estrogen-progestin is fully as effective as—if not slightly more effective than—estrogen alone. It should, therefore, be recommended for postmenopausal women for the prevention of heart disease. The other side of the coin, of course, is the possible increase in the risk of breast cancer in women on postmenopausal hormone replacement. This risk was defined in studies of estrogen alone, not combination therapy. We must await information on whether the estrogen-progestin combinations carry any risk of developing breast cancer.

This might sound like a complicated issue, and until now the decision of whether or not to take hormones after menopause has been terribly confusing for many women. For the first time, though, we have more solid information that will help women make a smart, customized choice. The decision of whether to take hormones should be approached like solving an equation. On one side of the equation are the benefits; on the other, the risks of hormone therapy. These risks and benefits will vary from woman to woman, depending on her personal chance of getting various diseases. In general, the benefits of hormone treatment (including a lowered risk of heart disease and slightly greater life expectancy) diminish the longer the hormones are taken. On the flip side of the coin, the risks—such as possible increased risk of breast cancer—climb with long-term hormone use. Here's how the equation pans out.

For most postmenopausal women, especially those with one risk factor for heart disease (such as smoking, hypertension, diabetes, or a sedentary lifestyle), the benefits of hormone replacement outweigh the risks. This holds true even for women with a first-degree relative (a mother or sister) with breast cancer. However, the equation shifts for women with no risk factors for heart disease and two first-degree relatives with breast cancer. For these women, hormone replacement therapy carries more risk than benefits. Other important factors to put into the equation include one's risk of bone loss (hormones protect bone density) and one's symptoms associated with menopause (hormones reduce hot flashes and other unpleasant sensations).

And more recently, a new factor must be added to the equation—that is, the impact of hormones on mental functioning. It has been suggested that estrogen may protect against Alzheimer's disease, the most common form of dementia and one of the greatest fears of older people. If further research confirms that estrogen protects the brain, then this will prove to be a serious factor to include in any woman's decision about hormone replacement.

Aspirin

Aspirin has many beneficial effects. It is a potent agent in "thinning the blood," that is, making it less likely to clot. It has the negative side effect of intestinal bleeding and therefore should be used with caution. Attempts have been made to use aspirin's blood-thinning properties to help prevent heart attacks and other vascular problems, such as stroke, in which development of blood clots plays an important role. In one major study of women aged thirty-four to sixty-five years, those who took between one and six regular aspirin tablets (325 milligrams each) per week had a 32 percent reduction in the risk of heart attack when compared with those who took no aspirin. Studies of men have yielded conflicting results. While one study of men aged forty to eighty-four showed a 40 percent reduction in heart attack risk with regular aspirin use, another study showed no such benefit. When the results of all the studies are combined, aspirin appears to be useful in the prevention of heart disease in men. Several other pertinent studies are currently underway.

What to do? Unless you have a reason not to take aspirin (for instance, you have a bleeding ulcer or you're taking other anticoagulants, such as coumadin), one baby aspirin (162 milligrams) per day seems a reasonable choice for all older people. If you take aspirin, which we recommend, remember you are taking a potent blood thinner! Make sure to clear any regular aspirin use with your doctor.

Antioxidant Vitamins

Interest in antioxidant vitamins such as vitamin C, beta-carotene, and vitamin E in preventing heart disease stems from their possible role in blocking the effects of low-density lipoproteins (LDL—the "bad cholesterol"). In a dietary survey and follow-up of nearly 40,000 American men age forty to seventy-five years, those with higher intakes of vitamin E had fewer heart attacks. Men who take vitamin E supplements have one-third as many heart attacks as those who do not, and postmenopausal women with high vitamin E in their diets have a lower risk of death from heart attack than those with low vitamin E intake. While one recent study has suggested that higher blood levels of beta-carotene may be associated with maintaining memory in old age, the results are still too sketchy to warrant a firm recommendation for their regular use. Other important studies have yielded conflicting results, however. It is simply not clear whether antioxidant vitamins reduce the risk of major diseases. Among smokers, carotene intake reduced the risk of heart attacks while it had no effect on nonsmokers, and 200 mcg per day of selenium may offer protection against lung cancer and perhaps other cancers as well.

As with many aspects of research in nutrition, further work is needed in this area. However, for the present, the bulk of the available research suggests for older persons there is likely benefit and no risk to daily vitamin E supplements of at least 200 IUs per day, more than can generally be found in multivitamins. It is likely that you need to take this for at least two years before there is a benefit.

Homocysteine and Folic Acid

Over the past several years, we have learned that a high blood level of homocysteine, an amino acid, represents a very significant risk factor for the development of vascular disease (including both heart attack and stroke). Elevated homocysteine carries as much risk as hypertension. The first hint came with the recognition that individuals with homocystinuria—a rare genetic disorder in which blood homocysteine reaches astronomical levels—develop severe vascular disease in adolescence, and in some cases even in childhood. Twenty years ago the first scientific reports appeared linking moderately elevated levels of homocysteine in individuals who did *not* have homocystinuria with premature development of heart disease and stroke. Recently the relationship between homocysteine and vascular disease has come under close scrutiny, and we have dramatically increased our knowledge of this important risk factor. Blood homocysteine increases with age and with the number of cigarettes smoked, and is higher at all ages in men than in women. Higher homocysteine levels are also found in individuals who have hypertension, high blood cholesterol levels, and a sedentary lifestyle. Thus high homocysteine levels appear in individuals with generally unfavorable cardiovascular risk profiles. The higher one's blood level of homocysteine, the greater one's risk of vascular disease. High homocysteine levels have also been associated with reductions in some mental functions, which are presumably related to the presence of vascular abnormalities in the brain.

In a very important recent development, we now know that blood homocysteine levels are highest in individuals with low dietary intakes of folic acid. Folic acid (in the form of folate) is widely found in normal diets, and is especially rich in uncooked leafy vegetables, liver, and fruit. Meat, dairy products, cereal, and flours are also good sources of folic acid. A recent report from the Nurses Health Study, which included data from 80,000 nurses followed for fourteen years, showed that those with higher dietary folic acid intakes are at decreased risk of developing heart attack. Supplementation of the diet with folic acid reduces homocysteine and presumably decreases the subsequent risk of vascular disease. These findings have spurred the recent national movement for the supplementation of food such as bread with folic acid to assure adequate folic acid intake in the broad population.

We recommend that older individuals supplement their diets with 400 mcg of folic acid daily. As is discussed elsewhere (chapter 6), supplementation with folic acid may expose some individuals with coincident vitamin B12 deficiency (which occurs in approximately 1 in 20 older persons) to development of neurological disorders. This can be avoided by additionally supplementing the diet with 1mg of vitamin B12 (cobalamin) daily. If there is any question regarding the presence of vitamin B12 deficiency, which is most common in older people with stomach disorders, individuals should consult their physicians before regular supplementation of their diets with folic acid.

In addition to the relationship between folic acid, homocysteine and the risk of vascular disease, an important relationship also appears to exist with homocysteine, vascular disease, and vitamin B6, another essential element widely found in most diets. Deficiency of vitamin B6 is more common in the elderly, particularly those with high alcohol intake. Recent studies suggest that increases in vitamin B6 intake in the diet also reduce the risk of heart attack, thus providing support for supplementing the diet with several milligrams of vitamin B6 daily.

STROKE

Stroke, a devastating disease that interrupts brain function, takes two basic forms—ischemic and hemorrhagic. In ischemic stroke, blood vessels in the neck or brain become clogged, either from a blood clot or with cholesterol-laden plaques like those that develop in the heart in patients with coronary heart disease. With hemorrhagic stroke, a brain vessel bursts, leaking blood into the surrounding brain tissue.

The most effective prevention for stroke in older persons is aggressive treatment of high blood pressure. We have known for some time that treatment of hypertension in older persons with elevated systolic *and* diastolic pressure reduces the risk of stroke. Now we know that this is also true in the case of isolated systolic hypertension. The age-old advice that elevations of systolic pressure alone reflect "normal aging" is archaic and simply wrong. The benefits of treating isolated systolic hypertension hold for all older people, including those over eighty years of age, and for both men and women of any race. Proper treatment for ISH is inexpensive and safe.

Smoking cessation is also effective in decreasing the risk of stroke. In the case of heart disease, the benefits accrue regardless of the age at which you started smoking or how heavy your habit was.

While there has been much discussion, and some research, regarding the impact of physical fitness on the risk of stroke, we don't know for sure whether there is a meaningful connection between the two. Thus, no specific recommendations can currently be made in regard to exercise and the risk of stroke.

OSTEOPOROSIS

In both men and women, bone strength gradually declines after the third decade of life. In women not taking estrogen replacement therapy, this age-related thinning of bones markedly accelerates after menopause. The term osteoporosis refers to bone loss exceeding that associated with normal aging, which is so severe as to place an individual at significant risk for bone fracture. While osteoporosis is a very common and important disorder in older people, and increases fracture risk, it does not by itself cause fractures. Fractures have many causes, including such factors as loss of muscle mass and strength (sarcopenia), and disorders of balance and mobility which boost the incidence of falls. This is a critical issue in the health of older people, as falls are the major cause of fracture. Older individuals rarely suffer a fracture without a fall or some other trauma.

The most common fractures in older individuals are in the hip, spine, wrist, and ankle. Repair of hip fracture requires major surgery. While death from hip fracture has fallen dramatically over the past decades, and now is in the range of 10 to 15 percent, this remains a very serious medical emergency in older persons. In the United States, it is estimated that there are 250,000 hip fractures in older persons per year, with 80 percent occurring in women. Most people with hip fractures can regain the ability to walk after intensive rehabilitation, but others become totally dependent as a result of the injury.

Fractures of the spine usually take the form of the collapse of vertebrae, which may lead to severe back pain, exaggeration of the curvature of the spine, and loss of height. This is the cause of the "shrinkage" many older people notice in their late seventies and eighties. Fractures of the wrist (Colles's fracture) usually occur when an individual stretches out an arm in order to break a fall. These fractures are generally easily managed surgically, though complete recovery may take months. Ankle fractures commonly occur in older people following the kinds of twisting injuries that might cause nothing more than sprained ankles in younger people.

Detection: It is important to emphasize that it is only valuable to screen for osteoporosis (or any disease in an older individual) if one intends to act on the results of the screening test. If it is unlikely that an intervention would be used if an individual is found to have a low bone density, there is no point in undergoing screening tests, no matter how efficient, sensitive, or inexpensive they may be. Thus, an older physically active healthy man with no evidence of a bone disorder or fracture and who is not in a high-risk group (i.e., not a heavy smoker) would not ordinarily be considered a candidate for screening. Similarly, a healthy, physically active postmenopausal woman who has been taking hormone replacement therapy since the beginning of menopause and has no risk factors or clinical evidence of osteoporosis does not require screening.

So who should be screened, and how? Two approaches for screening for osteoporosis are available. The first, simple X-rays, are not sensitive enough to detect mild or even moderate bone loss and thus are of very limited value in screening. Of much greater value is the Dual Energy X-ray Absorptiometry test, called DEXA for short. This method is fast, accurate, precise, relatively inexpensive, and not associated with high radiation exposure. It has become the gold standard for measuring bone density. Using this technique, bone density can be measured at multiple sites, including the wrist, hip, and spine—the most common sites for fracture. Such screening is recommended for anyone at very high risk for osteoporosis (see below) or for those considering hormone replacement therapy to evaluate their risk of fracture. Medicare provides coverage for bone density examinations for postmenopausal women.

Prevention: Several factors increase the risk of developing osteoporosis. One very important factor is postmenopausal loss of the hormone estrogen, which helps protect bone density. As bone density declines with age in women, fracture rates rise dramatically, especially in the eighth and ninth decades of life. Caucasian women have a higher incidence of osteoporosis than African Americans, who generally have greater bone density at all ages. Women of slight build are at greater risk for osteoporosis, perhaps because heavier people place added stress on their bones, which is thought to help maintain bone strength. Smoking is a major risk factor for accelerated bone loss with aging. Sedentary people, especially those immobilized for long periods due to illness, have significant bone loss. Men deficient in the hormone testosterone are at risk for significant bone loss at any age. And individuals whose diet is deficient in calcium, or who suffer from intestinal diseases which limit calcium absorption from the diet, are also at higher-than-average risk for developing osteoporosis.

As with many aspects of "usual aging," the risk of osteoporosis can be reduced significantly by regular physical exercise, as discussed in chapter 6. And smoking cessation should be a first line of defense. Beyond exercise and smoking cessation, the intervention most effective in preventing osteoporosis among women is hormone replacement therapy.

HORMONE REPLACEMENT THERAPY

Hormone replacement therapy slows the accelerated rate of bone loss after menopause. The beneficial effects of estrogen on bones may be due in part to the fact that it increases growth hormone levels, which increases both bone density and muscle mass. Estrogen reduces the fracture rate in both those who have never had a fracture as well as those with prior fractures. Estrogen is effective given by mouth, or via a skin patch, regardless of the age at which it is initiated up until the seventies. However, the earlier it is started and the longer it is given, the greater the benefit in protecting bone. But estrogen is not without its risks. It may promote the development of cancer of the lining of the uterus and boost the risk of breast cancer. But estrogen does not erase the effect of other risk factors. At least one study has shown that postmenopausal women on estrogen who continue to smoke do *not* gain the protective effect of estrogens on bone density.

Calcium

Nutrition has an important impact on bone health, and it's never too late to improve your diet. That goes for reducing the risk of heart disease and some cancers by reducing fat in the diet—and in this case, increasing calcium intake to protect the bones. Calcium supplements slow age-related bone loss, not only at menopause, but even ten years after menopause, whether or not an individual's diet is low in calcium. A daily intake of calcium of 1200 mg is recommended for older people. Since healthy older people average

700–800 mg of calcium in their diet, supplementation of 500 mg of calcium daily—along with 700 International Units of Vitamin D3 (Cholecalciferol) to increase absorption of calcium from the intestines—decreases age-related bone thinning and the risk of fractures.

Beyond *preventive* strategies, a number of medicines and other approaches are available for the *treatment* of established osteoporosis. It is worth noting, however, that the potent biphosphonate drug alendronate (Fosamax) is being considered for chronic use as a preventive in women unable or unwilling to take estrogen. We discuss Fosamax below.

Vitamin D

Vitamin D helps strengthen bones; healthy older people should take 700 International Units daily in conjunction with dietary calcium supplementation of 500 mg (the goal is 1200 mg of calcium per day from diet, and if need be, supplementation as well). Alternatively, if you don't want to take pills, milk is an excellent source of both calcium and vitamin D.

Calcitonin

Calcitonin, a hormone that influences bone metabolism and can be administered either through a nasal spray or by injection, increases bone mineral density and decreases fractures of the spine and hip in people with established osteoporosis. This drug has been approved by the FDA for the treatment of osteoporosis, and is especially recommended for women who cannot, or should not, take estrogen. Anyone taking calcitonin must also take calcium supplements.

Biphosphonates

Biphosphonates, a group of medications which increase bone mineral density in the spine and decrease the rate of spinal fractures, have received a great deal of attention as of late. Two forms are currently available—etidronate (Didronel), the first available in the United States, and alendronate (Fosamax), released more recently. Fosamax is significantly more potent than Didronel. In general, the biphosphonates are effective in increasing bone strength and decreasing hip and wrist fractures. They are currently recommended only for individuals who have established osteoporosis and should be taken with both calcium and vitamin D supplementation.

Fluoride

Early on, fluoride appeared to offer substantial promise in the treatment and perhaps even the prevention of osteoporosis since it induced development of additional bone mass (most treatments only reduce bone loss). Unfortunately, the new bone created was found to be brittle and fracture rates actually *increased*. A new slow-release form of fluoride has been developed. When administered on a cyclical basis with calcium supplements, this new formulation reduces spinal fracture rates. But this cannot yet be recommended as a routine treatment for osteoporosis.

DEMENTIA

There is no such thing as senility. The view that old age is inevitably accompanied by substantial reductions in mental function is clearly wrong. In addition, the view that loss of mental function in old age is due largely to "hardening of the arteries" has been disproved. Growing old, for most people, means maintaining full mental function. This is not to say that many older persons do not suffer from loss of cognitive function, but age is not the sole causative factor.

The most common age-related changes in cognitive function are generally modest, and most often isolated to memory. This is sometimes referred to as benign senescent forgetfulness, and must be distinguished from the full-blown syndrome of severe cognitive impairment known as dementia. Current knowledge regarding the causes of age-related losses of mental function, and approaches to its prevention, are reviewed in chapter 8. This section will focus on current knowledge regarding strategies for the prevention of Alzheimer's disease and other forms of dementia.

Dementia, the most common form of which is Alzheimer's disease, is an extraordinarily important geriatric disorder because of its marked increase with advancing age, and the dramatic toll it takes in destroying quality of life and shortening life. It robs people of their personalities, their ability to interact with others, and to function effectively. It brings tremendous emotional and financial costs. Dementia is *not* normal aging, and probably afflicts only about 10 percent of individuals over the age of sixty-five.

MULTI-INFARCT DEMENTIA

Multi-infarct dementia develops as many small strokes and creates a progressive reduction in mental sharpness. It occurs most often in diabetics and those with widespread cardiovascular disease and long-standing hypertension. Treatment of all forms of hypertension helps prevent this kind of dementia. Some, but not all, studies suggest that there is a role for the hormone estrogen in reducing the risk of stroke. (Current information regarding the prevention of stroke is discussed earlier in this chapter.)

ALZHEIMER'S DISEASE

Most established risk factors for the development of Alzheimer's disease, such as a strong family history, history of head injury, and inheritance of certain forms of apolipoproteins, cannot be prevented. However, substantial interest is developing in three possible approaches to prevention: 1) postmenopausal hormone replacement; 2) administration of nonsteroidal anti-inflammatory agents

(NSAIDs); and 3) dietary supplementation with folic acid and vitamin B12.

Hormone Replacement

Researchers have found that Alzheimer's disease is slightly more common in elderly women than in men, and that estrogens appear to serve as nutrients for cells from the area from the brain most impaired in Alzheimer's disease. Estrogen deficiency is emerging as a possibly important risk factor for developing Alzheimer's disease. Some believe that estrogens might prevent, or delay, the onset of Alzheimer's disease. In one study, 1,100 elderly women (with an average age of seventy-four years) who were initially facing evidence of Alzheimer's disease were followed with thorough yearly examinations. Alzheimer's disease developed in 16 percent of those who had never taken estrogens, but in less than 5 percent of those who had taken postmenopausal estrogen treatment—a big difference. The likelihood of developing Alzheimer's disease was related to the duration of estrogen administration, and fell to less than 2 percent in women who had taken estrogen regularly for at least a year. While this extraordinary finding has added substantial fuel to the fire of investigations of hormone replacement therapy and Alzheimer's disease, it requires more scientifically rigorous follow-up studies. Despite the preliminary nature of these findings, this study provides substantial optimism that we may at last have found an effective prevention strategy for women at risk for this terrible, disabling disorder.

Nonsteroidal Anti-inflammatory Drugs (NSAIDs)

Nonsteroidal anti-inflammatory drugs include aspirin and several nonaspirin agents such as ibuprofen (such as Motrin, Advil, and Feldene). These drugs are commonly used for minor injuries and arthritis. Long-term use of NSAIDs seems to protect against the development of cognitive decline in older persons. But additional studies will be required before a cause-and-effect relationship can be developed, or specific recommendations promulgated for the value of nonsteroidals in the delay or prevention of Alzheimer's disease. Again, however, the early evidence is quite hopeful.

Vitamin Supplementation

There is a significant relationship between blood levels of folic acid and vitamins B12 and cognitive decline. Low blood levels of these vitamins are associated with high levels of homocysteine, which has in turn been implicated in the development of vascular disease, including coronary heart disease and low cognitive function. While definitive evidence is not yet available regarding this issue, special attention has focused on folic acid, which is readily available and inexpensive. Proponents suggest that everyone take 400 mcg of folic acid daily and even go so far as to advocate including folic acid as a supplement in ordinary foods, just as vitamin D has been included in milk. This issue requires further study, however, since such an approach is not entirely without risk. Folic acid supplementation may mask the presence of underlying vitamin B12 deficiency, which is fairly common in older individuals. It is likely to be some time before this debate yields specific recommendations regarding folic acid supplementation of foods. In the interim, individuals should consult their physicians as to whether folic acid supplementation is appropriate for them. And they should inquire as to whether they are at special risk for the development of vitamin B12 deficiency.

VACCINATION

Influenza Vaccine

Among the greatest advances in health promotion and disease prevention in older persons has been the development of safe, effective influenza vaccines. Influenza is an extremely dangerous, often fatal disease in older persons. In a nonvaccinated group living together, such as in a nursing home or in elderly housing, an influenza epidemic can sweep through the entire population very rapidly. Influenza infection circles the globe annually, and each year the offending virus differs from that of the preceding years. In most years, the change in the virus is modest and individuals previously immunized through vaccination or influenza infection are at risk for only a moderately severe illness, if they get sick at all. On occasion, a major shift occurs in the genes of the influenza virus. Such viruses enter a population without protective immunity and severe epidemics, such as the pandemic of 1918, ensue in which large proportions of the elderly population die.

Since the annual migration of influenza virus begins in the Far East months before the viruses arrive in the United States, a program has been in place for years in which the new strain of influenza virus is identified at the outset of an influenza outbreak in the Far East, and a vaccine developed which is available in the United States months before the expected local arrival of the virus. The vaccine is available in the late fall, and should be administered before the New Year to all elderly. While some individuals experience side effects, such as discomfort at the site of vaccination or a modest "flulike" illness with mild fever and general achiness, these symptoms are not very common, generally last only a day or two, and are not sufficient to avoid routine influenza vaccination in all elderly people every year. Medicare covers influenza virus vaccines for older people.

Pneumococcal Vaccine

Pneumococcal pneumonia is a common, serious, and occasionally fatal illness in older individuals. An effective pneumococcal vaccine is available and should be administered to everyone over the age of sixty-five. Unlike influenza virus, the offending agent in pneumococcal pneumonia, the pneumococcus bacterium, does not undergo a genetic shift annually, and thus one vaccination confers a long term of protection. Older individuals who received a pneumococcal vaccination prior to reaching age sixty-five (because they were at special risk for the development of pneumococcal pneumonia) should be considered for reimmunization if at least six years have passed since their first pneumococcal vaccination. Those who have had an organ transplant or who have certain forms of kidney disease are at added risk. Medicare covers pneumococcal vaccines for older people.

Tetanus Vaccination

Tetanus, while a relatively rare disease in older individuals, can be severe and is often fatal. Tetanus vaccination is very effective in preventing tetanus infection. Anyone who has received the typical full three-dose primary series of tetanus-diphtheria vaccination (DPT) should receive a booster every ten years.

CHAPTER SIX

THE ROLE OF EXERCISE AND NUTRITION IN MAINTAINING HEALTH

RELATIONSHIP OF PHYSICAL ACTIVITY TO HEALTH

Overall Survival

There is a simple, basic fact about exercise and your health: fitness cuts your risk of dying. It doesn't get much more "bottom line" than that. Couch potatoes are now being grouped with cigarette smokers as taking their lives into their own hands. The substantial protective effect of physical activity was found to persist even to advanced old age. For instance, when over 40,000 postmenopausal women were studied over a seven-year period, those who did regular exercise were 20 percent less likely to die than those who were sedentary. The more frequent the exercise, the greater the benefit, but you don't have to overdo it. Moderate exercise such as bowling, golf, light sports, gardening, walking, and the like proved to be nearly as protective as vigorous exercise.

Another important finding is that the benefits of exercise even go so far as to negate the adverse effects of other risk factors, such as smoking, high blood pressure, and high blood sugar! The most fit people, even if they smoke or have high blood pressure, are still at lower risk of death than nonsmokers with normal blood pressures who are couch potatoes. This dominant effect of fitness over other risk factors, and its apparent effect as an antidote for other risk factors, makes physical fitness perhaps the single most important thing an older person can do to remain healthy. Physical activity is at the crux of successful aging, regardless of other factors.

This protective effect of exercise brings to mind a colleague whose strength and vigor belie his age and abundance of bad health habits. This man is an excellent squash player, despite his large pot-belly and his smoking. It is apparent that his enhanced physical performance is decreasing his risk of early death and perhaps serves as an antidote to some of his other lifestyle foibles. This may be heretical to health promotion and disease prevention advocates who, of course, want everyone to maximize their health-promoting activities and minimize their risk factors. But if you are at risk because of certain habits that you cannot change, getting in good physical shape is one valuable step you can take to keep yourself alive longer.

KEEPING THE GAINS FOR A LIFETIME: WHAT IT TAKES

When you sum up the powerful effects of moderate exercise on the health of older people, it's hard to imagine why we aren't all out there working up a sweat. Fitness boosts strength; it cuts the risk of death; it improves mood and reduces the impact of other health risks. But keep this in mind: you have to use it, or risk losing it. In order to reap the benefits of physical fitness, you don't need to *get* in shape—you must *stay* in shape. Physical activity must be maintained for a lifetime. The requirements to maintain a level of physical fitness do not increase—that is, you do not have to work harder and harder to stay in the same place. In fact, just continuing your initial level of training is usually adequate.

Furthermore, the benefits of exercise appear to be cumulative, which is good news for those of us who can't, or won't, fit long exercise sessions into our busy lives. To reap the kinds of benefits we've been talking about, you need to burn about 150 extra calories a day—or 1,000 calories a week. But you can divide this up any way you wish. For instance, you can walk briskly for half an hour every day or you can walk for just ten minutes three times a day. The goal is to exercise on a regular basis at least several days a week. What you do and when you do it is up to you.

IMAGE VS. REALITY: PHYSICAL FITNESS IN OLD AGE

The traditional image of extreme old age is one of frailty, weakness, and physical inertia. Take the grandmother in her rocker as an example. The idea of her jumping up out of that chair and trading her knitting needle for a squash racket or her slippers for cleats is a cross between unthinkable and sadly amusing. The notion runs contrary to what we often expect of older people—and closer to home, what we fear most about ourselves. The couch potatoes among us likely fear we'll *never* be able to work up a good sweat right now, let alone when (or if) we reach our nineties. But as the MacArthur studies show, very old people—even those who have never exercised before—are capable of becoming more physically fit. And physical fitness enables older people to function better in everyday life, as well as to live longer and better even in the face of other health problems or bad habits. Even as time conspires to rob us of our physical strength, balance, and endurance, we can fight the clock. And many older people are winning that fight.

WHAT HAPPENS TO THE BODY AS WE AGE

Unless we take some action to the contrary, the older we become, the less physically fit we become. Thus the stationary grandmother of lore does, to some extent, reflect some unfortunate truths about what aging inflicts on the human body. Doctors refer to the physical ravages of aging on our muscles as "sarcopenia." Our muscles weaken and shrink; we begin to lose our sense of balance; we often walk in a slow, shuffling, unbalanced fashion; it becomes harder to breathe and use oxygen to nourish our bodies. The decline of physical fitness with aging does not magically develop at age sixty-five, but begins at middle age and progresses steadily thereafter. The steady decline is known as "usual aging." But that doesn't mean *you* have to age in the usual manner. The critical thing to keep in mind is that severe physical decline does *not* have to happen to you.

PHYSICAL DECLINE AND DAILY LIVING

To most people, the physical decline that accompanies aging is not so important on the basketball court as it is in regular daily life. Walking up stairs, reaching for a can on the top shelf of the kitchen, getting out of bed in the morning, dressing oneself—if we become unfit, all of these mundane tasks become more like chores as we age. For a seventy-five to eighty-year-old with a sedentary lifestyle, just taking a shower uses over 50 percent of his or her full strength. Small wonder that many older people become winded with even minor exertion, even if they don't have heart or lung disease. And women (whose muscular strength and lung capacity are, on average, less than men's at every age) are hit harder by the debilitating physical effects of "usual aging." At age seventy-five to eighty, women on average have an aerobic capacity 15 to 20 percent less than men of the same age. It is also important to note that when aging promotes a gradual physical decline starting in middle age, a terrible downward spiral often ensues. The experience of feeling weak leads us to become more sedentary, and this inactivity in turn leads to further frailty. It is this spiral that often leads to total dependence on others, loneliness, and isolation.

EXERCISE FOR OLDER PEOPLE

Our society and media are full of powerful contradictions, and the image of older people is no exception. While the grandmother in her rocker sits at one extreme, magazines and retirement community ads offer a sharply contrasting view. Picture the perky, silver-haired tennis buffs who appear on their covers, nary a hint of weak bones or sagging muscles. As usual, the truth is in a gray area somewhere in the middle of the two extremes. The average older person is not vigorous and does not participate regularly in golf, tennis, bicycling, or even walking. Nor is he necessarily confined to a rocking chair or wheelchair. The proportion of the population that participates in *no* leisure time physical activities—the couch potatoes—does, in fact, increase with advancing age. In the "young-old," those between sixty-five and seventy-four, one out of every three women and one out of every four men report no participation in leisure time physical activities. And in the "old-old" (seventy-five-plus years), a group more severely ravaged by the effects of disease, physical activity falls even more. Half of women and nearly 40 percent of men in the oldest age group are couch potatoes, and less than one in five participates in regular exercise. But this does not mean that all is lost. It just means it's time for a wholesale shift in the way we live our lives if we want to age successfully. And it's never too late to start. Even people in their nineties can start becoming stronger and functioning better every day.

Take ninety-one-year-old Edward as an example. Edward hardly exercised a day in his life until age eighty-six. That's when he arrived at the Hebrew Rehabilitation Center for the Aged and needed something to do to fill his time. He signed up for an exercise program, "Fit for Life," focused on weight training in older people. Despite a serious case of peripheral neuropathy which robs his legs of a great deal of feeling, Edward does three sets each of eight leg presses (about 150 pounds), knee extensions (about 50 pounds), leg curls (about 70 pounds), and chest presses (about 75 pounds) three times a week. He does the leg presses one leg at a time because of the problems with his legs. "It doesn't make any difference how old you are, you can get stronger and better. Once I started, I felt better, stronger," he recalls. "Once you get going, you're full of action. The weight lifting helps my walking, I feel better, I sleep better, I eat better. It has changed my life." Edward had to purchase a new suit for a recent occasion, as his chest had become too bulky for the old one. He hadn't gained a pound—just a lot of muscle.

TURNING BACK THE CLOCK: HOW TO SLOW THE CHANGES OF AGE

The frailty of old age is largely reversible. Most older people, even the very old and weak, have the capacity to remarkably increase their muscle strength, balance, walking ability, and overall aerobic power. What does it take to turn back the aging clock? It's surprisingly simple and the research has proved that it has little to do with how old you are or what shape you're in at the start. The key is to exercise regularly, and the amount you do, plus the intensity and duration of the activity, are what make all the difference. Success is determined by good old-fashioned hard work.

What kinds of activities make a meaningful difference? Both aerobic exercise and so-called resistance training (weight lifting) offer important benefits to older people. Let's take a look at the effects of each type of exercise.

AEROBIC EXERCISE

Aerobic activities such as calisthenics, rapid walking, jogging, dancing, hiking, and the like increase flexibility and overall endurance or aerobic power, but not strength. Several important research studies have shown that older people can increase their general physical fitness—that is, their heart and lung fitness—with regular aerobic exercise. In many cases, the improvements exceed those seen in younger adults, and the results are that many older persons who regularly participate in endurance exercise are more physically fit than their sedentary middle-aged counterparts. This certainly surprised the researchers. And the added good news is that these aerobic activities are safe for older people, cause few injuries, and even fewer major adverse health consequences. Furthermore, it doesn't take long to see the positive results. After less than a year of regular exercise (e.g., walking several days a week for forty-five-minute sessions), older people increase their overall fitness dramatically—in many cases doubling their endurance.

Weight Training: Pumping Iron

You probably think of weight lifting or other strength training as a young person's sport. But that's a stereotype we must erase, because weight training can make a tremendous difference in older people's strength and overall ability to function. Strength or "resistance" training increases the size and strength of muscles without improving endurance. Even the "oldest-old" respond well to resistance training. Their muscles grow in size and strength much as younger people's do. What's required for success? Just as with aerobic exercise, the critical factor is not your age or initial strength, but the frequency, intensity, and duration of your training. Again, the harder you work, the better you do—even in the face of physical impairments.

Consider the case of eighty-nine-year-old Irving, who started exercising for the first time at the age of eighty-seven, also in the "Fit for Life" weight-training program. Today, he is more physically active than he's been in years. Irving uses all five weight machines in the gym—leg presses, leg extensions, leg curls, chest presses, and the triceps machine. He trains three times a week, and does three sets of eight repetitions on each machine. Even though his macular degeneration has rendered him nearly blind, he uses his hands to feel for the knob to set each machine. And the increased strength and balance imparted by the weight training has enabled him to take part in many other vigorous life activities. "I dance with women when the band is here. I dance Tuesdays and Thursdays. I walk east to west in the building ten times before breakfast. I walk straight instead of shuffling. I used to go side-to-side. Doing physical fitness gives me the energy to dance, to sing. It gives me lots of energy. My family can't believe it." Irving's trainer, Evelyn, notes that the weight training also has a powerful impact on self-esteem and self-confidence. She believes that the strength training produces the spontaneity and energy needed to take part in many other stimulating activities, like dancing. And the competitiveness among her ninety-plus iron pumpers, she reports, is just as heated (and fun) as that in a young person's gym.

Sara, ninety-one, knows that weight training can make a dramatic difference even when physical disability impairs your ability to move and function normally. After she fractured a hip and had a stainless-steel pin inserted for support, Sara had a great deal of trouble walking. Her weight-training program, which consists of either leg presses or leg curls three times a week, has brought her back to the point where she can walk a quarter of a mile without assistance and pump the pedals on a stationary bike. "I feel better physically and mentally. Inside and out I feel wonderful. I feel I must go for that exercise three times a week, I must. You have to push yourself." And push herself she does. Sara now can take fifty pounds of pressure on the leg curl machine and a startling 150 pounds of pressure on the leg press. Her workout consists of a quarter-mile walk to the gym, then three sets of leg weights, ten repetitions each, and then a quarter-mile walk home.

OTHER BENEFITS OF WEIGHT TRAINING IN OLDER PEOPLE

Weight training makes a meaningful difference in the lives of older people in several ways. And to give you an idea of how fast the benefits accrue, consider the findings of one important study: after just three months of training, older men doubled the strength of their quads (the large muscles in front of the thigh that straighten the knee) and tripled the power of their hamstrings (the large muscles in back of the thigh that bend the knee). It is important to note that these muscles not only got bigger, but significantly stronger as well. Individual muscle fibers enlarged, and more protein appeared in the muscles—two key measures of improved muscle quality. In other words, as we like to say, the muscles didn't just get juicier—they got meatier. In fact, over the course of the training, strength increased 5 percent with each training session! Studies have also looked at nutritional supplementation in addition to weight training in older people. The results: muscles got bigger, but not stronger. Exercise alone does both critical jobs.

And there's more good news—this time both for vanity *and* good health. Contrary to popular belief, we now know that pumping iron can help you lose weight. People commonly think that only aerobic exercise has this important effect. But science has shown that by turning up the metabolism of muscles (that is, making your body's engine burn a little harder every day) you burn more calories. And that translates into lost weight.

Finally, in addition to boosting strength and burning calories, weight lifting may offer a third powerful benefit to older people's health. Studies have shown that even short-term weight lifting can help reduce depression in older people. This could be extremely important, as depression is epidemic in our society and terribly prevalent in older people.

Pumping Iron in the Nursing Home

You might be wondering just who these older iron pumpers actually are—that is, do they resemble real people, or are they more like the mythologically active seniors on the magazine covers. The answer will probably surprise and please you. One of the important studies on senior weight lifters looked at the oldest, weakest nursing home residents and found that they, too, could become stronger, more fit, and better at everyday tasks. Their balance improved, they learned to walk more quickly and steadily, climb stairs, and so on. These gains in turn decreased their risk of falling and sustaining fractures and other injuries.

The studies involved frail older people up to ninety-eight years of age who live in a long-term care facility. Three times a week for eight weeks, these people did three sets of exercises on traditional weight machines, with eight repetitions each set. They did the following ten exercises: 1) the biceps machine to strengthen the upper arm muscles which are used to flex the elbow; 2) shoulder exercises to strengthen the upper arms and shoulders; 3) knee extensions to work the quadriceps muscle at the front of the thigh; 4) the triceps I machine to strengthen the muscles at the back of the upper arm which extend the elbow; 5) the triceps II machine to strengthen those same muscles in back of the upper arm; 6) plantar flexors to strengthen the ankle and muscles in back of the calf; 7) hip flexors to strengthen the muscles that bring the knee toward the chest; 8) knee flexors to strengthen muscles in back of the thigh; 9) hip abductors to strengthen the muscles at the sides of the hips and thighs which pull the legs out to the side; and 10) hip extensors to strengthen the muscles in the buttocks and lower back. The results were astounding. Muscle strength increased 174 percent on average, and the walking speed of individuals increased by 50 percent. Two of the participants in one study actually began to walk without the assistance of canes. The results set in quickly—and the study participants were able to retain their newfound function with just one weight lifting session per week. This proves that you don't have to become an Olympic athlete to have real, meaningful improvements in your quality of life and health.

And yet despite powerful scientific (and anecdotal) evidence of how much weight training can help older people, resistance exercise is largely neglected in the elderly. Ageism is such that there is something unsettling or odd about the concept of legions of older persons pumping iron. Old-age weight lifters are few and far between. Fewer than 7 percent of men and 3 percent of women participate in any form of iron pumping—and when you look at the "old-old," those figures fall to 5 percent for men and 1 percent for women. How sad, when you consider that these exercises make a tremendous difference in daily life, and that injuries and other health problems are quite rare in properly supervised programs. Hopefully, as the word gets out, these numbers will change.

Risks of Exercise

They say the bad often comes with the good, and like anything else, exercise is not without its risks. Happily, they are few and usually minor. There are two main types of injury—minor muscular/skeletal problems and major heart-related health problems.

Minor muscular/skeletal injuries are fairly common, including such things as pulled muscles, or worse still, a torn Achilles tendon; slipped intervertebral disk; collisions with exercise equipment; falls and overuse problems that lead to ankle and knee injuries; and so on. The injury rate is one in twenty for walkers age seventy to seventy-nine. This is much lower than the rate among joggers: 57 percent. Most of these injuries are minor and get better on their own, without medical attention, however. Overall, supervised regular exercise programs are exceptionally safe for older people and significant injuries are particularly uncommon.

Next: heart problems. You've no doubt heard stories about trained athletes and even marathon runners dropping dead while exercising. This is mainly a problem for people with significant, unknown underlying heart problems who participate in sudden vigorous exercise without a doctor's okay. The secret to success is to have a thorough medical evaluation and to participate in *supervised* exercise programs if you are at added risk. Everyone known to have heart disease or to have multiple major risk factors such as diabetes, smoking, or hypertension, and all individuals over age sixty-five should have a thorough medical evaluation prior to initiation of regular exercise programs. But remember: even if you have an underlying heart problem, as many older people do, your doctor can help you find an exercise program that is safe for you and that will help you improve both your overall condition *and* your cardiovascular health.

PHYSICAL FITNESS AND THE RISK OF SPECIFIC DISEASES

We've talked about the tremendous value of exercise in boosting overall health. But exercise can also be used to reduce the risk and complications of specific health problems. Of course, exercise is not a panacea: there is still controversy about the role of exercise in preventing common diseases such as breast and prostate cancer and stroke. But physical activity can make a major difference in the risk of some diseases.

Coronary Heart Disease

Beyond doubt, physical activity cuts the rate of coronary heart disease. The greater the "dose," the greater the effect. The more physical activity you participate in, the lower your risk. Couch potatoes are 80 percent more likely to develop coronary disease than the most active people.

High Blood Pressure

Exercise cuts the risk of *getting* hypertension in half, and also helps lower existing high blood pressure. And just as in the case of overall conditioning, a little exercise goes a long way. Even moderate amounts of physical activity reduce blood pressure in people with hypertension. But while exercise does produce meaningful reductions in blood pressure, it rarely solves the entire problem on its own. Medications and other treatments may be needed in addition to physical activity to bring blood pressure into a desirable range. Physical activity should be considered as an important *adjunct* to the treatment of hypertension, not as a sole remedy.

Colon and Rectal Cancer

The bulk of scientific evidence shows that an increase in physical activity protects against colon cancer—but *not* against rectal cancer.

Diabetes and Related Problems

Many older people have what's known as "type 2" or non-insulin-dependent diabetes. This form of the disease is generally treatable with diet and oral medications rather than with insulin injections. By age sixty-five, about 40 percent of the population has high blood sugar and many have a condition known as Syndrome X, or insulin resistance syndrome. This is usually accompanied by a large potbelly, high blood pressure, and high blood fats. What does all this have to do with exercise? Physical activity cuts the risk of all these health problems, thereby cutting the risk of heart disease and stroke—major killers of older Americans—in turn. And many people are surprised to learn that both weight lifting *and* aerobic exercise help reduce these risks. For many years, aerobic exercise alone got all the credit.

Arthritis

Many people believe that exercise *causes* arthritis by placing stress on the joints. But in fact, moderate regular exercise often *relieves* arthritis pain and disability—particularly the pain of osteo-arthritis and rheumatoid arthritis. These days, exercise is used as a key tool in the treatment of severe arthritis. And again, both aerobic and resistance exercises are helpful.

Osteoporosis

Osteoporosis, or loss of bone density, is a major cause of dis-ability in postmenopausal women. It can lead to painful and even life-threatening fractures. Weight-bearing exercise such as walking, dancing, or lifting weights has long been viewed as a potential means of counteracting the age-related reduction in mineral density that occurs after menopause. The hope was that exercise would protect bones and decrease the likelihood of fracture. However, despite the substantial amount of research in this area, the jury is still out on the value of exercise *alone* in thwarting the age-related reduction in bone strength. We believe that physical activity offers some benefits, and that the more intense the activity, the greater the gains. But to keep up a running theme, a little goes a long way. One recent study in women aged fifty to seventy found that bone density increased in both the hip and spine with twice-weekly strength training over the course of a year.

Falls and Balance

There is more to preventing fracture than reversing age-related reductions in the strength of bones. In general, you don't fracture your hip if you don't fall. While physical activity, including both aer-obic and resistance exercises, may be of value in improving bone strength, it may make an even greater contribution by improving balance and strength, and promoting the ability to walk and climb stairs without assistance, thereby cutting the risk of falls. The equation is a simple one: exercise equals better strength and balance, which equals fewer fractures. And happily, variety is the spice of life: studies have shown improvements with such diverse activities as strength training and Tai Chi Chuan in older people.

NUTRITION IN OLD AGE

It's well known that many children eat poorly, replacing milk with soft drinks and trading their sandwiches for candy at school. But many older people eat poorly as well—for a variety of reasons. A combination of long-term bad habits, sometimes poverty, dental problems, and often lack of knowledge about the nutritional requirements of aging all play a part.

For most older people, the same general nutritional guidelines proposed for younger adults continue to make sense. There are, however, some specific age-related changes that healthy older persons should be aware of and that might change one's nutritional requirements over time.

Calories

Over time, aging men and women progressively lose muscle mass, which means that it takes fewer calories just to live and function normally. The so-called basal metabolic rate, that is, the energy we use to perform basic body functions, drops by about 10 percent by the age of seventy-five years. Add to that the fact that older people are less physically active and the result is substantial decline in the caloric needs of older adults. This means that you either have to eat less to maintain your weight or exercise more so you can consume the calories you're used to having.

Water Balance

An important aspect of overall nutrition is water balance. Several factors conspire to put older people at a relatively high risk of dehydration. For example, older people have a lesser capacity to conserve water through the kidneys, as well as a significantly lower sensation of thirst. This is particularly troublesome in the face of acute illnesses with fever, such as common colds and flu, which push the risk of dehydration even further. In fact, dehydration increases the risk of flu-related complications (such as sinusitis and pneumonia) in older people. Older people should consume about one and a half to two quarts of fluid per day. This need not be consumed as water alone. Juices and other beverages that consist mainly of water are fine choices as well.

Recommended Dietary Allowances and Dietary Reference Intakes

Relatively little is known about the effects of age on requirements for specific nutrients. Recommended dietary allowances (RDAs), promulgated by the Food and Nutrition Board of the U.S. National Academy of Sciences since 1941, define the level of essential nutrients adequate to meet the known nutrient needs of practically all healthy persons. RDAs were designed to avoid nutrient deficiency and associated diseases. RDAs are provided for protein, eleven vitamins, and seven mineral and energy requirements. Currently the RDAs are being replaced by Dietary Reference Intakes (DRIs), a term that encompasses the former RDAs as well as issues such as tolerable upper intake levels. Also, in a major advance, DRIs are being developed for various age groups, including separate recommendations for ages 51 through 70 and over 70.

Fat

Older people should follow the same guidelines for fat intake as younger people are given: that is, no more than 30 percent of total daily calories from fat, with no more than 10 percent from saturated fat, 10 percent from polyunsaturated fat, and 10 percent from monounsaturated fat. Since cholesterol does not seem to carry as much risk for the elderly as in younger adults, limitation of cholesterol intake does not seem necessary in most older persons.

Carbohydrates

Dietary carbohydrates, sugars and starches, often found in "white" foods, i.e., sugar, potatoes, pasta, and bread, should supply 55 to 60 percent of daily calories. Unfortunately, most people get no more than 45 to 50 percent in their diets. The emphasis should be on complex carbohydrates, which contain soluble fiber and are found in some fruits, peas, beans, and lentils. These can help reduce the incidence of constipation and formation of another gastrointestinal problem known as colonic diverticuli. Dietary fiber also reduces blood fat and sugar levels, and may be important in preventing heart disease.

Protein

Older people may need more protein than younger people. Protein is found in meats, fish, poultry, eggs, and dairy products. Approximately 12 percent of your total calories should come from protein. While the average American diet contains more than this amount, many elderly do not eat enough protein because of their inability to chew or afford meats, or inability or lack of desire to cook. Infections, surgery, and metabolic stresses, all relatively common in older people, also increase protein requirements. Chronic dietary protein insufficiency may reduce the ability to fight disease and heal wounds, and may cut one's overall muscle strength.

VITAMINS

Vitamin B6

Many older people are deficient in vitamin B6, which can impair one's ability to fight disease, and can lead to increases in homocysteine, a risk factor for heart disease and stroke discussed in chapter 5. Good dietary sources of B6 are chicken, fish, kidney, liver, pork, eggs, and to a lesser extent unmilled rice, soybeans, oats, whole wheat products, peanuts, and walnuts.

Folic Acid and Vitamin B12

Folic acid and B12 intake in older adults is a topic of great interest. One of the most common changes that affect nutrition in old age occurs in the gastrointestinal tract. Atrophic gastritis, a wearing out of the lining of the stomach leading to lower levels of acid secretion, is seen in approximately 35 percent of men and women by age eighty. This problem leads to decreased absorption of folic acid and vitamin B12. Other factors, such as poverty and use of many medications, are also associated with poor folic acid intake in older people.

Folic acid (or folate) is found in a wide variety of foods—leafy vegetables, liver, yeast, and some fruits. Still, many older people have low blood levels of this important nutrient. Low or even low-normal folic acid levels are associated with yet another health problem—that is, high levels of the amino acid homocysteine, which is a risk factor for heart disease and stroke, and possibly dementia (see chapter 5).

Vitamin B12 deficiency among the elderly is also common, and is associated with anemia, neurologic disorders, and other major health problems. Low intake of red and organ meats, major dietary sources of vitamin B12, is an important risk factor for vitamin B12 deficiency among poor elderly adults.

We believe that all older people should take supplements of at least 400 mcg of folic acid per day. Routine use of folic acid may carry some risk, however. About one in twenty older people suffers from vitamin B12 deficiency, a condition that can lead to irreversible nerve damage. Folic acid will mask the anemia of B12 deficiency, and it is this anemia which usually brings the B12 deficiency to medical attention. To minimize this risk, consult a physician before beginning routine folic acid supplements. Dietary supplements of 1 mg of vitamin B12 for each 400 mcg of folic acid will also be effective in treating most cases of B12 deficiency.

FAT-SOLUBLE VITAMINS

Vitamin D

In general, the elderly should be at *lower* risk of deficiency in fat-soluble vitamins—A, D, K, and E—because of their ability to store these vitamins in the liver and fat tissue. But vitamin D deficiency is common in older people for several reasons. You get vitamin D both from foods and from sunlight exposure, and homebound or institutionalized elderly have limited dietary intake and often lack adquate sunlight exposure. Good dietary sources of vitamin D include fortified milk, butter, eggs, and seafood. Vitamin D is important in increasing the absorption of calcium from foods, and the combination of vitamin D (700 International Units daily) and calcium (500 mg daily) supplements daily has been shown to strengthen bone and decrease the risk of fracture in healthy elderly people. Try for a total of 1200 mg/day of calcium, most from diet, and if need be, add supplements.

Vitamin K

Vitamin K deficiency is rare in the absence of certain medications, especially antibiotics. Vitamin K is required for the regulation of blood clotting, and the best dietary sources are green leafy vegetables, but small amounts exist in milk, dairy products, meats, eggs, cereals, and fruits. Elderly persons in good health are not known to have increased need for vitamin K.

Antioxidants—Vitamins A, C, and E, Beta-carotene, and Selenium

In the aging process, so-called free radicals are considered enemy number one. Free radicals are the result of normal oxygen metabolism in the body and are thought to cause damage to cells throughout the body. Studies have shown a strong association between free radicals and many diseases that are associated with aging, such as cardiovascular disease, cancer, cataracts, macular degeneration of the retina in the eye, and changes in the immune system. The body's natural defenses against these toxic compounds may falter over time or under stressful conditions. That's when free radicals can accumulate and cause damage. The possible heroes of this story are the so-called antioxidants. Some vitamins and minerals, especially vitamins C, E, beta-carotene, and selenium, are thought to save the day by acting as scavengers of these free radicals. It's an exciting premise and a great story line, but one that needs further study.

Vitamin A and Beta-carotene

Vitamin A is stored in the liver and is important in vision and the healthy immune system. Dietary sources of vitamin A include liver, fish, liver oil, whole milk, eggs, carrots, and dark leafy vegetables. So far, we've focused mainly on vitamin and other nutrient *deficiencies.* But in the case of vitamin A, older people need to worry not about getting too little, but about getting too *much.* The elderly are at risk for vitamin A *toxicity* because it is easily absorbed, tends to build up in the liver, and produces toxins which are slow to clear out of the body. The elderly should *not* take vitamin A supplements. Symptoms of acute vitamin-A toxicity include headache, drowsiness, dizziness, irritability, nausea, vomiting, and diarrhea. Symptoms of chronic toxicity include skin disorders, disturbed hair growth, fatigue, and enlarged liver and spleen.

Beta-carotene, a chemical precursor of vitamin A, is a different story. Some say that beta-carotene protects against certain cancers and cardiovascular disease, and may help with maintenance of memory. The jury is still out on this topic, however.

Vitamin E

Vitamin E is another fat-soluble vitamin categorized as an antioxidant. The richest sources in the diet are common vegetable oils and the products made from them, margarine and shortening. Vitamin E is also found in wheat germ, nuts, and green leafy vegetables. There is no consistent evidence for different vitamin E requirements with age. Neither deficiency nor toxicity is common, as vitamin E is ample in normal diets and adults can tolerate very large amounts without symptoms.

Dozens of studies have recently been published supporting the association between high intake of vitamin E and lower incidence of coronary artery disease in middle-aged women. In one report, patients with documented coronary artery disease who used vitamin E supplements for two years had a lower risk of death due to cardiovascular disease and a lower risk of heart attack.

Vitamin E has also been shown to enhance immune function in older people—and not just those who are frail, sick, and malnourished, but healthy older people as well. Interestingly, more is *not* necessarily better. Supplementing a normal diet with 200 mg of vitamin E per day seems more effective than using 800 mg per day.

Vitamin C (Ascorbic Acid)

Vitamin C, plentiful in citrus fruits, berries, peppers, potatoes, and tomatoes, has been linked to a reduced risk for cancer, cataracts, and coronary artery disease.

Vitamin C deficiency is associated with poor wound healing, easy bruisability, and the disease scurvy. There is no evidence that vitamin C requirements are greater in the elderly. Supplementation with very large doses (greater than 1,000 mg per day) may cause kidney stones or chronic diarrhea.

Recent evidence suggests that *low* blood levels of vitamin C are associated with memory loss in older people, but this requires further study. There is little support for a role for vitamin C in prevention of viral illness, or the common cold. And finally, there is conflicting evidence surrounding vitamin C and the risk of cardiovascular disease, cancers, and eye diseases.

MINERALS

Selenium

Selenium is a mineral with antioxidant properties and has been shown to be essential for health. Foods with the highest concentrations include fish, especially tuna, and several vegetables, including asparagus. Brazil nuts are loaded with selenium, and meat, poultry, and bread are other food sources. Geographical studies suggest that areas with higher soil levels of selenium have lower incidences of cancer mortality. This information prompted a decade-long study which looked at the effect of selenium on skin cancer. While the incidence of skin cancer was not reduced by selenium, daily supplementation of 200 mcg *per day* was associated with a 50 percent reduction in total mortality and significant reductions in the incidence of lung, colorectal, and prostate cancer. While it is too early for a general recommendation to supplement the diet with selenium, so far the information is encouraging and side effects seen, minimal.

Requirements for most minerals do not change with age, with the exception of iron and possibly calcium. Iron requirements in healthy, well-fed elderly women are lower than those for younger women. This is because after menopause, women stop losing blood each month, which means they lose less iron. Yet despite this decreased need for iron, iron deficiency is still common among older people, and is probably due to both poor dietary intake and decreased absorption in the stomach and intestine. The best-absorbed form of iron is in meats, but iron is also available in eggs, vegetables, and fortified cereal.

Calcium intake in elderly adults was fully discussed in the section on osteoporosis (see chapter 5). Good dietary sources include dairy products, broccoli, kale, collards, and some calcium-fortified foods. The recommended calcium intake for older men and women is 1200 mg per day. As the usual diet of older people includes only 700–800 mg of calcium daily, supplementation with 500 mg of calcium, along with 700 International Units of vitamin D3, is recommended to retard age-related bone loss and prevent fractures. For those who don't like taking pills, milk is an excellent source of both calcium and vitamin D.

AGING SUCCESSFULLY: WHAT YOU CAN DO FOR YOURSELF

We have entered a new era of health promotion and disease prevention in older persons. This exciting era is one in which there is as much, or more, that we can do for ourselves than even our doctors can do for us. The remarkable and rapidly emerging scientific evidence reviewed in this chapter spurs tremendous optimism for the powerful benefits of exercise and nutritional interventions in preventing or delaying chronic diseases in late life. And most important, eating well and working our bodies will likely provide extra years of productivity, health, and high function.

We leave you with Anne, age seventy-four, who understands the real bottom line about the dramatic role exercise and good diet can play in later life: feeling *well*. A self-described couch potato in her youth, Anne now has an exercise regime to rival most women a fraction of her age—and this despite painful osteoarthritis diagnosed more than thirty years ago. Her routine is as follows: three times a week, she swims for one mile, which takes about fifty minutes. On off days, about two to three times a week, she rides a recumbent bike for thirty-five to forty minutes. On the cycling days, she also weight trains, doing leg lifts, leg presses, lateral pull-downs, and many other exercises. She works on all twelve machines in her gym, setting the weight as high as eight ten-pound plates for some leg exercises. Finally, she does yoga once a week for an hour, with stretching, balance, breathing, and relaxation exercises. "I have less pain because of the exercise. You get so used to it, if you don't do it, you don't feel good. When I don't exercise, I feel crabby, logy, not myself. My feeling is, if I didn't exercise, I might be in a wheelchair."

CHAPTER SEVEN

BEYOND EXERCISE:

Strategies to Maintain and Enhance Physical Performance in Old Age

T HE MACARTHUR RESEARCH Program in Aging revolution-
ized the study of physical performance in old age. Prior
studies of physical function in older individuals were often
limited to identifying serious physical limitations, such as trouble
feeding, washing, dressing, shopping, using the telephone, washing
clothes, and so on. The trouble is, this means that more than two-
thirds of older people were excluded—and lumped into a category
of "not-disabled." Our goal was twofold. First, we aimed to measure
physical performance in the elderly, looking at a comprehensive
range of activities that go well beyond minimum function. And second, we wanted to identify the factors that promote sustained and
perhaps even improved physical function in healthy older people.
Both goals were met, and some of the new information proved
important and surprising.

Most people assume that physical exercise and other fitness-
oriented activities are the main routes to good physical function in
old age. But physical fitness is just one of many important factors.
We were surprised, in many ways pleased, to learn that mental ability and social relationships were also critical factors in determining

older people's physical status. The link between mind and body is a powerful one.

The MacArthur Study evaluated over 4,000 older people from East Boston, Massachusetts, Durham, North Carolina, and New Haven, Connecticut. The study participants represented typical older Americans. They varied in age from seventy to seventy-nine years, with an average age at the outset of the study of just over seventy-four. Nearly half had incomes under $10,000 a year, 19 percent were African American, more than half had less than a high school education, and 17 percent reported less than an eighth-grade education. The researchers identified the top third in terms of mental and physical function; we call them "successful agers."

These older men and women were asked a wide variety of questions, including their basic demographic information (age, race, and so on); behaviors (diet, exercise, smoking, etc.); social network (whom they count as friends, close relatives, etc.); and psychological characteristics (self-esteem, happiness, and so on). And among dozens of other tests and measurements, the study participants were given a series of tests to measure physical performance, such as the ability to use their hands, arms, trunk, and lower extremities. Their balance and gait were also evaluated. Gait was measured in a test of the speed of walking, and to assess balance skills, individuals were timed on how long they could stand on one leg or hold a "tandem stand," that is, a position in which one foot is held straight in front of the other, heel to toe. An additional test measured how long it took to stand up from sitting in a chair and sit down again five times without using the arms for support. To measure fine physical performance, a test of manual ability and handwriting was also included. Several tests of mental function were given, and those results are discussed in the next chapter.

At first blush, some obvious characteristics of "successful physical agers" appeared. They tended to be male, white, relatively affluent, better educated, and healthier than those who aged less well.

But more important, we wanted to determine those factors that help predict *future* successful aging—that is, enhancement or maintenance of physical and mental abilities. This requires long-term follow-up, and indeed, the older people in this study were re-examined three and eight years after the initial testing.

Some of the factors we discovered were quite interesting and unexpected. More predictable were such factors as age (i.e., those in their early seventies were more likely to increase their physical functions than were older people); having an income of over $10,000 per year; having high lung function at the outset (presumably a measure of physical fitness); being male; being of normal weight; and participating in *either* moderate or strenuous physical activity. Moderate physical activity, such as leisurely walking or gardening, was every bit as strong as strenuous exercise in predicting later physical ability.

Much more surprising, though, is the fact that those who had higher *mental* function are also more likely to retain *physical* function than others. And another striking finding, new to the medical literature, was that the frequency of *emotional support* was a very strong predictor of the likelihood of enhancing physical function over time. Social support, as we discuss in chapter 10, comes in two forms: so-called instrumental support, such as cooking meals, shopping, and cleaning; and emotional support—being there for other people to support them psychologically, to cheer them up and talk over their problems. The MacArthur Study found that it was the frequency of *emotional* support, not *instrumental* support, which was the powerful predictor of maintained and even enhanced physical function with age. Just good, old-fashioned talk therapy from friends and loved ones helps to keep the aging body vital.

The most striking finding was that nearly a quarter of these successful agers further improved their function over the eight years studied, and more than half maintained their previous high level of function. This dramatic finding clearly debunks the myth that losses in physical function are an inevitable part of advancing age. Now, for the first time, our challenge is to take the blueprint of successful physical aging provided by the MacArthur Study and apply it to the lives of all older people.

CHAPTER EIGHT

MAINTAINING AND ENHANCING MENTAL FUNCTION IN OLD AGE

WHEN OLDER MEN and women are asked about their hopes and aspirations, they name their primary goal—to remain independent and continue to take care of themselves. Similarly, when they are asked about their greatest worries, they stress the fear of becoming dependent on others. Loss of either physical or mental function is a major threat to independence, and almost all older people have relatives or friends who have, however reluctantly, become dependent because of such deficits.

The greatest dread for many older people is Alzheimer's disease, the debilitating form of dementia which receives tremendous publicity these days. Misplaced eyeglasses or struggling for the right word might just irritate a younger person. But for the elderly such errors bring to mind the looming threat of Alzheimer's disease or other permanent mental disability.

In this chapter, we review the research answers to four key questions about mental function that are of most concern to older men and women:

    1. How worried should older people be about decreasing mental function?

2. Are cognitive losses an inevitable part of aging?

3. Can decreases in mental function be prevented?

4. Can older people increase any of their mental abilities?

HOW WORRIED SHOULD OLDER PEOPLE BE ABOUT DECREASING MENTAL FUNCTION?

The fact is, older people worry excessively about losing mental ability. Living in a nursing home is one indicator of decreased functional level, either physical or mental. But only 5 percent of people over the age of sixty-five live in nursing homes, and that percentage has been falling for at least ten years. Ninety-six percent of older people are "community dwelling," as the Census puts it; they live in private homes, usually on their own or with family. Among those community-dwelling elders, fewer than 5 percent say that they need help in the basic activities of daily living, such as dressing, bathing, and eating. More than 95 percent take care of these things for themselves. Independence in such efforts means that these people are functioning mentally as well as physically. It does not mean, of course, that they have the same mental ability they had when they were younger. And it certainly doesn't mean that they are unconcerned about maintaining their functional level.

Fears of cognitive loss, and especially of Alzheimer's disease, are widespread among older people. And those fears are understandable. Alzheimer's places great burdens both on patients and those who care for them. It is also difficult to diagnose with certainty, except by analysis of brain tissue after death. Specialists believe, however, that cognitive tests and clinical examinations enable them to make a diagnosis with 90 percent confidence. Estimates vary, but it appears that about 10 percent of people over the age of sixty-five may have Alzheimer's disease. The proportion increases with age, however. At least one study suggests that among the "oldest-old," people aged from eighty-five to 100 or more, 30 to 50 percent may have some degree of Alzheimer's disease.

Nevertheless, one reassuring fact remains: even though the proportion of older people in the population has been increasing, and despite the fact that the relative increases have been greatest among the "oldest-old," the usual pattern is that older people maintain a good portion of their independence and mental sharpness.

We talked to some of the MacArthur Study "successful agers" about how they sustain their mental ability as they age. Many say they actively work on keeping their minds sharp, using a variety of mental games and exercises, or just keeping engaged in regular conversation.

Ernest, a MacArthur successful ager, finds that old-fashioned talk and reading keep his mind young. "I go to people's homes, they come to mine. We talk for one to two hours. We talk about current events. It's positively important. We keep up with the events of the day whether we like them or not, say they're great or ridiculous. I read a lot, I go to the library and the guys give me twenty or twenty-five books; if I read three of them, I'm doing fine. I read mysteries, I read nonfiction and fiction. I keep my mind busy."

Another successful ager, Allescio (age eighty-two), uses daily word games to challenge his mind and keep it running smoothly. "I do all the crossword puzzles and other puzzles in the paper every single day. I don't skip it. Every day without fail I do this to keep my mind active. I don't sit in a chair and watch TV." Vera, eighty-seven, takes a similar approach: "I do a lot of reading, play bridge three to four times a week, do crossword puzzles every day. I play Scrabble once a week, and another game of cards, pinochle, with someone else."

Others say that their daily occupations keep their minds active and young. They speak of keeping so busy, there's no opportunity for the mind to become dull. Clara, eighty-three, finds that helping tend her son's coin appraisal business and keeping her daughter's life in order has the added benefit of keeping her own brain alive. "I sit and count coins, check coins, and take care of the phones three days a week. No TV in the day—I've got things to do. I try to take care of everything in my home. I write everything myself—write letters to my sister and niece. And I baby-sit for my grandchild once a week overnight and take care of my daughter's dog. There's something doing all the time. I say you only go around once."

ARE COGNITIVE LOSSES AN INEVITABLE PART OF AGING?

To listen to the MacArthur successful agers, one might say no. The actual answer to this question is yes *and* no, or perhaps "yes, but . . ." Some mental processes do slow down significantly with age, but many do not. And as with many other characteristics of aging, the losses tend to be exaggerated, both by impatient young people and by older people themselves. Even older people who are reassuringly free of cognitive disease may feel that they are slowing down mentally and that they have trouble learning or remembering new things.

What are the mental differences between young and old? As a rule, older people do less well than younger ones on memory tests. However, most of this apparent effect of aging is caused not by aging itself, but by differences in health and socioeconomic status. Older people who are in good physical health, who have more years of education, higher income, and who are employed do better in memory performance than other elders.

One major study looked at how the mental function of a large group of people changed over a period of twenty-eight years. The study looked at several measures of mental function including the ability to use words and numbers accurately, to see the relationships between different shapes, and to draw appropriate conclusions from sets of facts. In general, there were no significant losses in these mental abilities before age fifty. Beyond that age, many older people lost some mental ability. But even in the oldest group, half of all people showed no mental decline whatsoever during the seven-year period from age seventy-four to eighty-one. Over the twenty-eight-year period, however, average decrements are substantial for all cognitive functions. One central goal of the MacArthur Study was to determine just what factors enable some people to retain their mental ability with age. We'll discuss those factors later in this chapter. The next challenge, of course, will be to develop tools to enable others to achieve that same success.

Another important issue is what happens to *elite* mental function with advancing age. For instance, does scientific or artistic achievement decline in any way? The answer is yes, but the age of peak achievement varies for different fields. Scientific creativity peaks earliest in the most abstract disciplines—mathematics and physics, for example. In biology, geology, and other fields that are less abstract and closer to "real-life" phenomena, the scientific peak comes at a somewhat later age. History and philosophy seem to be more age-tolerant pursuits. Overall, peak achievement in these varied fields averages in the late thirties or early forties.

But again, there is significant variability among different individuals. These differences are large, and at least as interesting as the averages. Just consider Michelangelo in old age, working at the top of crude scaffolding to paint the glorious ceiling of the Sistine Chapel. And to jump ahead a few centuries, Picasso, too, exemplifies sustained artistic achievement in old age.

Speed of Information Processing

But there are some negative facts about the aging mind that must be acknowledged. Two underlying brain functions do decline with age, for reasons that appear to be intrinsic to the aging process itself. The first is the *speed* of information processing and the second is certain kinds of memory. The first of these is well established; as the brain ages, the rate at which it can receive and process information slows. The reasons for that mental change are not well understood. One might consider cognition as a kind of computation process in a brain network consisting of billions of cells. As the brain ages, some of the links in that network are broken. As a result, information processing in the aging brain requires some neurological "detours" and these add to the time required to react. However, this does not necessarily cause functional impairment, since most activities of daily life do not test the limits of our ability to process information rapidly. And, more important, the speed of information processing is only one element in cognitive function; it is not the single, or even the most important measure of intelligence.

Furthermore, many older people tell us that when mental pursuits are important enough, one can compensate for minor changes in mental function with added patience and diligence. Charles, eighty-three, acknowledges that his mental speed may have slowed somewhat: "I keep thinking in the old days I could have gotten a thing done two weeks earlier." But he continues to pursue intellectual goals nonetheless: "So much depends on what your goals and values are," he stresses. "For me and my colleagues, who have been doing intellectual academic research all our lives, to suddenly give up and go sit in the sand or whatever would be psychologically devastating. To give up like that if you really have things you want to do—devastating." Charles finds that new technology gets in the way as well: "I used to have an excellent secretary and dictated everything, so I never learned to type. Now I'm learning to use the computer and to type, and I do all my work on the computer. This adds to the problems." But in spite of technological barriers and slight functional decline, the work excites him enough that he refuses to give it up. And MacArthur research suggests that this is part of a cycle that promotes mental ability: the more you have, the more you do; the more you do, the more you preserve.

Memory

The other underlying cognitive ability that reduces as we grow older is a certain kind of memory. Older people have some reduction in what is called explicit memory, which involves the intention to remember, and the subsequent ability to recall a specific name, number, or location on demand. Many older people find themselves racking their brains for a name or word that is well known to them, but which refuses to come to mind on demand. This reflects the reduction in explicit memory.

Other kinds of memory, however, show little if any decline with age. When things previously seen or heard are presented again, older people recall and recognize them about as well as young people. Perhaps most important, something called working memory, the learned routines on which all of us rely in our daily lives, shows little decline with age.

Older people do differ from young people in the conditions they require for effective mental performance. Many elders watch young people study for examinations or do math problems while listening to loud music or even lying on the floor in front of a booming television set. They may do quite well doing several tasks at once. Older people often cannot perform so well under these distracting conditions. We now have some clues to explain these generational differences. Older people are more distractible, less able to filter out stimuli that are irrelevant to the task at hand. Rather than giving up on a group of challenging tasks, elders would be wise to focus on one project at a time.

A triple message emerges from all this information. First, only a few specific cognitive losses appear to be caused by the aging process itself. Second, in this as in many other characteristics of aging, there are great differences among older people. Third, cognitive ability or intelligence, as it is usually called, is not one thing. Cognitive ability should be thought of in the plural, and not all cognitive functions age in the same way or at the same rate. For this reason, even moderate declines in some areas of mental functioning do not necessarily interfere with the ability to function or remain independent.

CAN DECREASES IN MENTAL FUNCTION BE PREVENTED?

There is no single preventive formula that enables people to avoid or minimize cognitive decline in old age. Many factors contribute to this much-desired outcome. Some of them are genetic, and thus beyond the control of the individual. Some are the result of early experience and opportunity, and are thus no longer controllable in old age. Most encouraging, some factors that minimize or avert cognitive loss can be undertaken at any age. We'll examine each category.

Genetic Factors in Cognitive Function

The relative importance of genetic versus environmental effects is best estimated by comparisons of adult twins who were reared apart. Dozens of adoption and twin studies, involving more than 10,000 pairs of twins, show that about half of all individual differences in general mental ability is determined by genetic factors. And this strong genetic effect on mental function persists in old age, even past the age of 80. While the impact of genes on mental function is greater than on some other characteristics, there is still substantial room for nongenetic (e.g., lifestyle) measures to improve mental ability.

Enduring Properties of the Person

The MacArthur Studies of Successful Aging (described in detail in the preceding chapter) found that people who are better educated, physically active, have good lung function, and high "self-efficacy" (which is related to self-esteem) are most likely to maintain sharp mental ability.

Education

Education was the strongest predictor of sustained mental function. People with more years of schooling are more likely to maintain high cognitive function. The continuing impact of education nearly fifty years after most of the study participants finished school suggests two possible effects. First, education early in life may have a direct beneficial effect on brain circuitry, which in turn enables the maintenance of cognitive function in old age. Second, education may set a pattern of intellectual activities—reading, chess, crossword puzzles, and the like—and this lifelong exercise of cognitive function serves to maintain it.

Lung Function and Physical Fitness

As part of their annual physical examination, many people are instructed to take a deep breath and blow through a tube as hard and as long as they can. The result of this strenuous exhalation, measured by machine, is known as the pulmonary peak expiratory flow rate. This rate is a strong predictor of mortality among older people—the better it is, the greater their chance of survival. It is also an indicator of cardiovascular fitness, which in turn is correlated with physical and cognitive function.

We were at first surprised by the MacArthur finding that older men and women who engaged in strenuous physical activity in and around the home were more likely to maintain their high cognitive function. We knew that exercise helped maintain *physical* function, but why did it also help maintain *cognitive* function? One possible answer came from a MacArthur laboratory experiment which measured the effects of exercise on the brains of adult rats. Increasing exercise caused corresponding increases in a chemical substance (nerve growth factor) which promotes growth of new brain cells.

This finding suggests that exercise enhances the function of the central nervous system, especially its memory function.

Self-efficacy: The Can-Do Factor

The fourth key factor that emerged from the MacArthur research as helping to sustain mental ability is an aspect of personality known as "self-efficacy." Self-efficacy is a person's belief in his or her own ability to handle various situations. It is the belief that one can solve specific problems, or meet specific challenges, and otherwise influence the course of events in one's everyday life. Many studies have shown that this form of self-esteem leads to improved performance of many kinds, including persistence in solving cognitive problems, success in mathematical performance, and mastery of computer procedures.

A sense of self-efficacy is particularly important for older men and women, who often falsely conclude that even modest age-related losses in physical ability must lead to drastic reductions in activities. Self-efficacy also has an impact on memory. Older people with low self-efficacy are more likely to believe that memory is a biological ability, and that it reduces inevitably as people grow older. Older people high in self-efficacy are more likely to view memory as a set of cognitive skills that, to some extent at least, can be learned and improved. The belief that memory is controllable in turn raises motivation and encourages effort. And to complete the loop, successful effort reinforces the underlying sense of self-efficacy. On the flip side of the coin, believing that memory is *not* controllable leads to resignation, lack of effort, and the downward spiral of unused abilities.

Environmental Influences on Cognitive Function

For most adults, the job is probably the single most important source of cognitive demands. And for many people, it is also the main source of mental stimulation. Remember the old adage "We become what we do"? People whose jobs promote self-direction, use of initiative, and independent judgment tend to boost their intellectual flexibility—that is, their ability to use a variety of approaches in order to solve mental problems. On the other hand, workers in routine and monotonous jobs working under close direction from a foreman or supervisor tend to lose intellectual flexibility.

The key point is that complex environments provide a variety of stimuli, choices, and opportunities, which in turn exercise and sustain mental function. The work situation is a major source of environmental complexity (or the lack of it), but paid work is not the only source. Similar effects have been shown for substantively complex unpaid work in the home and for students. And this is meaningful for older people, who often participate in unpaid work before or after official "retirement."

Just how work affects mental function is not yet known. It seems likely that practice makes perfect—that is, the continuous exercise of cognitive capacity in response to job demands has direct effects on problem-solving abilities. This can be thought of almost as a regular mental "workout." In addition, complex, self-directed work often leads to increased participation in intellectual leisure-time activities.

CAN OLDER PEOPLE INCREASE ANY OF THEIR MENTAL ABILITIES?

Yes. In the absence of major disease, memory and other cognitive functions can be improved in old age. Most of the methods require individual effort, however; there is not yet a magic cognitive pill to be swallowed.

Biomedical Approaches

Vitamin E, because of its antioxidant properties, has been advocated as a possible preventive of cognitive loss. More recently, research has begun to show positive effects of the female hormone estrogen on cognitive function in women. Estrogen seems to empower brain cells in several ways—by boosting their chemical function, stimulating their growth, and protecting them against toxins. The result, according to early trials, is improved memory, both in healthy older women and female Alzheimer's patients. In one small experiment, five out of six women who had mild Alzheimer's disease and wore an estrogen patch for two months improved in verbal memory and attention. Future research, in addition to validating this early work, must look for ways of obtaining the benefits of estrogen without its serious disadvantages (which include increased risk of certain cancers and feminizing effects on men).

As discussed in chapter 5, should further research confirm these early findings of estrogen's positive effect on the brain, the balance will likely be tipped in favor of estrogen replacement for many women who are conflicted about whether to take hormones after menopause. Improved mental ability will have to be weighed, along with improvements in heart and bone health, against potential risks of hormone replacement.

Training and Practice

Older men and women can improve their cognitive function significantly by means of appropriate training and practice. Elderly people who showed a clear decline in inductive reasoning (the ability to draw appropriate conclusions from a set of facts) and spatial orientation (seeing the relationships between different shapes) achieved substantial improvement after only five training sessions. Follow-up testing showed that these cognitive improvements were sustained.

Memory losses among healthy older people are also reversible with training. One study looked at the number of words people could recall after they had been presented briefly with a long random list of words. Before training, older study participants recalled fewer than five words from the list. Younger participants did better, which demonstrates the expected age-related losses in memory. Both the old and young experimental subjects then went through five training sessions in methods of recall. For instance, they were taught to group words into meaningful clusters, rather than trying to remember individual words out of context. And they were trained to link words to spatial locations or sequences already known—for instance, when trying to remember what groceries are needed, they might walk through the kitchen, where their minds would be triggered to remember the needed items.

When they were retested after training and practice, older people more than tripled their word recall, to about fifteen words. The memory performance of older people was thus not only much better than their own pretraining scores; older people with training also did much better than young people without training. Young people with training, however, did better still. Many people are amazed to learn that elderly men and women who have experienced some cognitive decline can, with appropriate training, improve enough to offset approximately two decades of memory loss.

Social Support

Continuing close relationships with others—family and friends—is an important element in successful aging. The mutual exchange of social support that goes on in these relationships has a positive impact on many aspects of physical function in older age. And now, MacArthur and other research shows that such support can also improve mental performance in older people. An experiment in a nursing home compared mental performance under three conditions in which the kind of social support varied. Nursing home residents were assigned randomly to three groups, each of which had the same task—completion of a simple jigsaw puzzle. All three groups had four twenty-minute practice sessions, followed by a timed test session. People in the first group were given verbal encouragement by the experimenter during practice—"Now you're getting it . . . that's right . . . well done." People in the second group were given direct assistance—"Are you having a little trouble with that piece? Let me show you where it goes." People in the third group were given neither assistance nor encouragement during practice. In subsequent tests, people who had been encouraged improved in speed and proficiency. People who had been directly assisted did less well than in practice. And people who had been left alone neither improved nor deteriorated.

There is a double lesson here. First, social support can improve the performance of certain mental tasks. Second, to achieve those improvements, the kind of support must be appropriate to the situation and to the needs of the individuals. We can only speculate on the frequency with which well-meaning or impatient younger people do things for their elders that they could do for themselves, and thus promote increasing helplessness and dependence instead of continuing function. The performance loss may be more a matter of lowered self-confidence and motivation than poor intrinsic mental ability. But the effect on performance is no less profound. The lesson for children of older people is clear: be patient, be supportive, but resist the urge to do things for your parents that they can do for themselves.

Increasing Self-efficacy

A sense of self-efficacy is a person's belief that he or she can deal with specific activities or problems appropriately, and with a reasonable prospect of success. When experience in a variety of situations confirms this belief, the sense of self-efficacy tends to broaden—and the person gains a readiness to face new problems and accept new challenges. Increasing self-efficacy for any activity, be it verbal memory or the high jump, requires a gradual series of experiences which begin at the person's initial level of confidence and comfort. It is important to provide clear evidence of success, with appropriate encouragement, and congratulatory feedback. Success at each level is followed by presentation of a slightly greater challenge. This same approach is used with remarkable success in the treatment of phobias, from air travel to snake handling.

When experiments are done to increase cognitive performance by means of increased self-efficacy, however, elders are less responsive than younger people to the experience of their own success. For example, after brief training in the use of memory aids, young adults are more likely than older adults to raise their trust in their own memory. Elderly men and women require more positive feedback than suffices for the young in order to see the same gains in self-efficacy. However, experiments with memory show that once older people are convinced of their ability, they devote more time and effort to the memory tasks, and thus attain further gains in both performance and sense of self-esteem.

WISDOM IN OLD AGE: BEYOND THE IMITATION OF YOUTH

That older men and women can prevent or even regain some of the cognitive losses that are usually and mistakenly considered an inevitable part of aging is tremendously encouraging. If successful aging is to be more than the imitation of youth, however, we must also ask whether there are valued human attributes that *increase* with age, or that might do so under appropriate conditions of opportunity and encouragement.

Thinking about this question leads us to ask what, beside the sheer passage of time, necessarily increases as one grows older. One answer to that question must be the accumulation of experience. Not all experiences are positive but, positive or not, the accumulation of experience continues as long as we live. Some experience becomes obsolete, of course, as the years pass. All of us "of a certain age," as the current phrase delicately puts it, have learned things that are no longer useful. One of us (RLK) knows how to start a car with a crank and how to do so without breaking his thumb, but for some considerable time there have been no opportunities to use that knowledge. Secretaries were once prized for skill at shorthand and accuracy at the manual typewriter, but those skills have been devalued by the tape recorder and the word processor. Past experience has also taught us things that are no longer true. Living through the years of the great economic Depression of the 1930s, for example, taught a generation to practice many small economies that are no longer necessary or appropriate. Are they valuable in some way nonetheless? Maybe so, maybe not.

Some kinds of experience clearly remain relevant, however. They are experiences that involve relationships with other people, human strivings and foibles, strengths and weaknesses. Knowledge in these domains, unlike technological competence, does not become obsolete. The heroes and villains of *Star Wars,* and the things that motivate them, are familiar to elders from the silent western movies that thrilled their childhoods on Saturday afternoons long ago. As we age, we can become wiser about ourselves and others, about the uncertainties of life, about what is ultimately important and unimportant in people's lives, about things that change and things that do not change in human affairs.

The idea that wisdom increases with age is not new. That belief was strongly held in many societies, but they tended to be societies in which technological change was slow and tradition was strong. Our own technology-driven society, despite nostalgic references to the golden years, tends to associate expertise with youth rather than age. But this is a partial truth at best, true for the technological sector, but not for the great domain of human affairs.

These ideas are admittedly speculative; little research has been done to test them. Recently there is increasing interest in doing so, however, and some interesting work is now under way. In the Berlin model of aging, wisdom is defined as the ability to exercise good judgment about important but uncertain matters in life. This ability involves both factual knowledge, which is often experience-based, and the use of that knowledge in reasoning and problem solving.

In experimental research using this model, people of different ages are presented with brief descriptions of difficult life problems and asked to discuss what they would do or advise if confronted with them. Here are some illustrative examples from the Berlin research and other sources:

Marian, a fourteen-year-old girl, has just learned that she is pregnant. What issues should she consider, what facts does she need, and what should she do?

A sixteen-year-old boy has been going with a girl of the same age for more than a year. He wants to get married soon. What issues should he consider, what facts does he need, and what should he do?

Joyce, a widow sixty years of age, recently completed a degree in business management. She had planned to open her own small business and has been looking forward to the challenge of doing so. She has just learned that her daughter-in-law has died, leaving her son with two small children. What should she consider in planning her own future? What additional information would you like to have in order to advise her? What should she do?

Sarah, now in her seventies and a widow, decided long ago to build her life around husband, home, and children. Her children are now adults with children of their own, all of them living far away. One day Sarah meets an old friend, also now widowed, who made a different life decision. She had a long and successful career, from which she is now retired, but chose not to have children. The meeting causes Sarah to think back over her own life. What might her life review look like? How might she explain her life choices to others? How might she evaluate her life?

The answers that people give to questions like these were rated according to the following five criteria of wisdom: 1) factual knowledge brought to bear on the question; 2) procedures and strategies for getting additional information; 3) recognition of long-term consequences of decisions; 4) sensitivity to religious and cultural issues; and 5) appreciation of the fact that no course of action is perfect—all have costs as well as benefits.

There is preliminary evidence that older people are among the top performers in responding to these kinds of questions. Unlike the case with short-term memory, for example, age-related cognitive deficits are not apparent in dealing with these lifelike problems. And although both young and old do best in dealing with life problems pertinent to their own age groups, for certain problems involving choices in later life, all of the top-rated responses came from older people. Also, elders did better than young people at problems that occurred at an unusual age. Finally, lest we be carried away by a vision of universal wisdom in old age, very few responses by people of *any* age were rated highly on all five of the wisdom criteria in the Berlin model.

CONCLUSION

The aging mind is, in many respects, a sound, flexible, useful mind. Fears of mental incompetence in late life, although they have some basis in reality, are often exaggerated both by young and old. In spite of age-related reductions in some mental functions, the vast majority of older men and women retain more than enough reserve capacity for meaningful and satisfying life, and for independence.

Later life is a time in which some men and women attain a degree of wisdom that only the thoughtful assimilation of long experience can confer. May it be so with the readers of this book.

CHAPTER NINE

MARKETING YOUTH: THE PILLS, POTIONS, AND LOTIONS OF ANTI-AGING

ONE MEASURE OF a society's perspective on aging can be drawn from its dollar expenditures on anti-aging remedies. The billions of dollars we spend on creams, pills, lasers, and other alleged high-tech and low-tech clockbusters gives us one clear clue: modern humans do not appreciate the look of old age. And millions of people trustingly shell out billions of dollars to erase it. Following are just a few of the most popular anti-aging products, what to believe about them, and what to reject.

DHEA

If we're to believe the promoters, DHEA is the closest we've ever been to discovering the fountain of youth. Many health food stores block their doorways with bottles and billboards announcing when the timebuster DHEA is in stock. The substance has been promoted as a panacea for everything from poor sex drive to early death. As usual, the truth lies somewhere in a huge gray area between cure-all and danger. DHEA may have some health benefits in certain people, but it carries serious risks as well.

DHEA is a hormone produced in the adrenal gland which is

then converted to both estrogen and testosterone. Blood levels of DHEA peak at about age twenty, then decline so that by age sixty they are one-third less those of young adults. Low DHEA levels are associated with age-related diseases and disorders, including cardiovascular disease, obesity, diabetes, some forms of cancer, osteoporosis, and dementia. Several studies have demonstrated a protective role for DHEA given to laboratory animals. So-called physiologic replacement doses of DHEA, that is, doses designed to increase blood levels to those in younger adults, have been claimed to improve immune function and possibly protect postmenopausal women from cancer. DHEA replacement also increases levels of something called "insulin-like growth factor," a substance which also declines with age. This suggests a possible mechanism for the relationship of low concentrations of DHEA to the increases in diabetes that occur in later life. DHEA supplements are also reported to improve physical and psychological well-being.

But the downside to DHEA is equally striking. High doses of DHEA can lead to liver damage. And because DHEA is a precursor for estrogen and testosterone, it could potentially promote cancers that are fueled by estrogen (such as breast and uterine cancers) or by testosterone (prostate cancers). This is especially worrisome because the amount of estrogen and testosterone the body makes after exposure to DHEA is highly variable, and there is no way to predict which patients will produce a large, potentially dangerous amount of estrogen or testosterone after taking DHEA. Beyond cancer, increases in testosterone may cause excessive facial hair growth in women, as well as changes in blood fats which might increase the risk of heart disease. The National Institute on Aging currently supports animal research of DHEA's "anti-aging" effects. But larger, scientifically rigorous human studies are needed to determine if there are benefits to this treatment, and to determine the type and severity of any side effects. DHEA is not currently approved for *any* indication by the United States Food and Drug Administration (FDA). We do not recommend its use at this time.

MELATONIN

Melatonin (scientifically known as N-acetyl-5-hydroxy tryptamine) is another of the highly hyped and wildly popular anti-aging "remedies." It is a hormone produced in the pineal gland, which lies deep in the brain. Normally, melatonin levels are highest during the night, and this hormone is considered important in induction of sleep. Melatonin levels fall with age, which may account for the high frequency of insomnia in older people. To date, most human studies using melatonin have been small and have lacked proper scientific controls. Melatonin appears to reduce jet lag symptoms in travelers. And in people with insomnia, nighttime doses of 0.3 to 1.0 mg appear to decrease the time needed to fall asleep and improve the quality of sleep. However, the dose sold in many stores—*without* a prescription—is 3 mg, which can lead to blood levels of melatonin forty times higher than normal. We do not know the short- or long-term effects of taking these higher levels, but some people experience drowsiness and headache the following morning.

Melatonin is also being touted as an anti-aging substance because of its antioxidant properties and because it may boost immune function. The National Institute on Aging is planning to support studies of melatonin's long-term effects and safety, but until more is known, we do not recommend its use as a long-term supplement. While melatonin has not been approved by the U.S. FDA, it can be purchased over the counter. Buyer, be patient: wait for more scientific proof.

HUMAN GROWTH HORMONE

Human Growth Hormone (hGH), which is produced by the pituitary gland in the brain, is yet another potential fountain of youth. It is available by prescription only. In young people, hGH is necessary for proper growth and development. Excess growth hormone secretion early in life, caused by pituitary tumors, can lead to excessive height. Excesses later in life, after growth has ceased, cause a syndrome termed "acromegaly," which is associated with hypertension and a variety of other tissue abnormalities. Many studies show a gradual reduction of hGH levels with aging so that about half of people age seventy years and older are partially or totally deficient in hGH. This hGH deficiency may be related to many physiologic changes in the older body, including decreased muscle and bone mass, and increases in body fat, specifically abdominal fat. As discussed elsewhere, an increase in the waist/hip ratio is an important risk factor for development of coronary artery disease.

Since hGH secretion is reduced with aging, the possibility exists that giving hGH might reverse or prevent some of the changes that occur with age. The findings on this score are mixed. Some beneficial effects of human growth hormone were demonstrated in a study of healthy men over the age of sixty. For six months, they were given doses of hGH designed to mimic normal levels in young men. The older men had an increase in muscle mass and skin thickness, a decrease in total body fat, and a modest increase in the amount of calcium in the lower spine. But a twelve-month follow-up study found that many of these positive changes started to reverse. Another more recent study of healthy older men found that while there were modest increases in muscle and decreases in fat, there were no improvements in functional ability, muscle strength, endurance, or mental function. The participants also experienced various side effects, which required a dose reduction. Finally, a study of sixty-six-to eighty-two-year-old women found that growth hormone promoted the development of increased muscle.

One very interesting discovery is that another chemical, called insulin-like growth factor, seems to be responsible for most of the benefits associated with growth hormone. The two work together in a kind of "hormone cascade," one triggering the other. This is potentially exciting news, because it's possible that down the road we might be able to give insulin-like growth factor *instead of* growth hormone, thereby avoiding the high cost and some of the risks of growth hormone. But this is still preliminary.

The National Institutes on Aging is presently funding five-year clinical studies at various centers throughout the United States to determine if growth hormone can help strengthen muscle and bone, and help reduce frailty in older people. Some of these studies combine hGH supplementation with both strength and aerobic training, since exercise has been shown to stimulate hGH secretion. Human growth hormone is exceptionally expensive, however—about $15,000 per year—and must be given by injection. And because excess hGH has significant side effects, such as diabetes, hypertension, nausea, and development of carpal tunnel syndrome, we recommend waiting for the results of these formal studies before having hGH injections.

Testosterone

There is substantial interest in the possible anti-aging benefits of testosterone, the male sex hormone. Testosterone levels fall gradually after middle age but "male menopause" is much more gradual than female menopause, and its severity varies widely from man to man. Testosterone replacement in castrated middle-aged men reverses declines in muscle and bone strength and sexual function. However, the relationship of low testosterone to the impotence that occurs in over half of men over age seventy is unclear. Testosterone administration generally does not improve potency in old age, since the causal factors are usually diseases, the effects of alcohol or medications, or psychological factors. The value of testosterone in increasing muscle strength and overall well-being in old men is not yet defined, though research is under way. There is substantial concern regarding the side effects of testosterone, including prostate enlargement and stimulating the growth of prostate cancer. At this point, not enough is known to recommend testosterone as an anti-aging form of hormone replacement therapy.

ANTI-AGING SKIN TREATMENTS

Of all the alleged anti-aging formulas and techniques, those designed to reverse skin aging are, as a group, the most popular and lucrative. The ubiquitous promises of cosmetics manufacturers to reduce "age spots" and erase other "unsightly signs of aging" are the logical and astonishingly profitable response to a society generally obsessed with resisting old age. But the language of these promises is flawed. In fact, what is generally considered the effects of aging on the skin is actually the result of sun exposure. These changes include wrinkling, a rough feeling to the skin, the loss of elasticity or sagging of the skin, the appearance of small blood vessels on the skin surface, and changes in the coloration of skin. These age/sun-induced changes, termed "photo-aging," occur mostly on exposed skin areas, such as the back of the hands, face, neck, and scalp. The most familiar signs are fine wrinkles around the eyes (crow's-feet), in front of the ears, and in the cheek areas; and coarse wrinkles, which are most prominent in the forehead (frown or worry lines), and around the mouth (smile and pucker lines).

One major category of anti-aging products includes cosmetics, which are intended to cover up the effects of photo-aging. Cosmetics are sometimes effective, and while they may make you look younger—and that may, in turn, make you feel younger—this should not be confused with actually modifying the aging process. It can be likened to sweeping the dust under the epidermal rug.

Beyond cosmetics, however, some anti-aging or antiwrinkle preparations promise not merely to disguise the ravages of age on the skin, but to actually reverse them. Some such antiwrinkle creams temporarily diminish the number or severity of fine wrinkles, but may actually be harmful to skin, and even worse, cause wrinkles over the long run. Such preparations cause mild irritation in the skin. The resulting inflammation and swelling stretches the skin, thereby removing minor wrinkles. When the short-term effect of the inflammation subsides, the original wrinkles reappear and the skin may have suffered additional damage. The result: greater wrinkling, or other adverse effects, in some cases.

TRETINOIN

Many well-designed studies have confirmed that the topical application of retinoic acid, in the form of tretinoin, or Retin A, reverses many of the effects of photo-aging in the skin. But severe photo-aging, such as deep wrinkles, respond much less well than mild changes. One landmark study demonstrated marked improvement not only in the *appearance* of the skin, but also in reversing underlying changes. This was proved with skin biopsies which were examined under a microscope. Since this initial study, many other large trials have confirmed that tretinoin application daily for several months reduces mild to moderate photo-damage in the skin—especially wrinkling—and can be helpful for mild changes in pigmentation such as liver spots. Significant improvement occurs in two-thirds to three-quarters of patients. Higher concentrations of tretinoin (0.05 percent) are more effective than lower amounts (0.01 percent). Improvements are seen not only in white patients, but also in those of Asian background. The longer tretinoin is used, the greater the benefits. Tretinoin is usually associated with mild side effects, however, such as irritation and inflammation of the skin, with reddening, some swelling, and discomfort. This occurs in approximately three-quarters of patients, but generally resolves after two to three months of continuous use, although it may signal a tendency toward longer-term side effects. Even after several years of continuous therapy, significant side effects have not been observed. Retinoic acid also has been shown to be effective in preventing or reversing the emergence or growth of certain forms of skin cancer, such as actinic keratoses, which are associated with sun damage. Retinoic acid should be prescribed by and used under the direction of a physician.

While the possibility has been raised that retinoic acid may have some generalized anti-aging effects beyond its value in reversing the effects of photo-aging, there are currently no scientific data to support this contention. Oral use of this agent for anti-aging purposes has not been studied, and is certainly not recommended.

AHA ACIDS

Alpha-hydroxy acids (AHAs), which include glycolic, lactic, or citric acid, are attracting increasing attention for their possible value in improving the status of aging skin. Recent studies have shown that the application of lotions containing glycolic acid to the skin of the forearm for six months reverses the age-related thinning of the skin. This is consistent with prior studies that have shown that AHAs can improve skin wrinkling. To date, these studies are too small in size and few in number to provide definitive information regarding the use of these agents to reverse signs of photo-aging. But substantial enthusiasm is growing, and more studies are underway. One attractive feature of the use of these agents is that they appear *not* to induce inflammation of the skin, a potential advantage over retinoic acid.

OTHER APPROACHES

Some claim that fish cartilage polysaccharide extracts are of substantial value in modifying aging skin. However, adequate studies of these compounds have not yet been conducted and at present they cannot be recommended.

But for people whose photo-damage to the skin is too severe for minor remedies like retinoic acid, there are other dermatological techniques available. These include chemical peels with agents such as phenol and trichloracetic acid, and dermabrasion, a physical technique in which superficial layers of the skin are scoured off to remove wrinkles. While these techniques are effective, their proper application requires substantial training and experience and there are significant potential side effects. They must be approached with great care, and conducted by a fully trained dermatologist or other physician experienced in the use of these techniques.

Also, laser treatment for the skin of the face is gaining popularity. The CO_2 laser is most commonly used, although the Erbium laser is coming into play as well. Laser surgery can reverse deeper wrinkles and more pronounced discolorations on the skin, such as liver spots—that is, conditions which peels or creams can't erase. However, the treatment is more costly and invasive than peels and other related treatments, and can cause major (weeklong) redness and oozing on the skin during the healing period. But many people are quite pleased with the results. Again, as with dermabrasion and the more potent chemical peels, it is critical to find a physician with ample experience and only choose the procedure if it is appropriate to your individual skin problem. These days, computer images can be used to predict likely "before and after" images. This can help patients bring their expectations in line with reality. For none of these procedures actually breaks the clock—at best, they just appear to turn it back a bit.

CHAPTER TEN

RELATING TO OTHERS

". . . only connect . . ."

A FEW YEARS AGO, a British film called *Howard's End* became deservedly popular in the United States. On the title page of the book on which the picture was based, just below the title itself, appear the two words quoted above: only connect.

No explanation is given and it is late in the book before the phrase reappears in the text. It comes as part of a climactic scene in which the heroine, middle-aged herself, confronts her older husband. Her demand is that he recognize himself—his own strengths and weaknesses—in the lives of others, including their misdeeds and misfortunes. She urges him to relate to others in ways that reflect that understanding and that offer support.

At that point we realize the ways in which the author, E. M. Forster, intended us to understand his brief injunction, only connect. It sums up his philosophy of life, his command for living, his sense of what it means to be truly human: connect with others, know what we have in common, help and be helped.

In the domain of human relationships, MacArthur and other research has validated, and in its own way deepened, the insights of everyday life. The linking of social relationships to longevity, the discovery that social support lies at the core of those relationships, and the special role of social support in aging have been gradually, but unmistakably, demonstrated. In this chapter we describe some of the main research findings in this area and the critical importance of connectedness in the lives of older people.

THE IMPACT OF SOCIAL CONNECTEDNESS ON HEALTH

We know four important things about the connection between social relations and health, and all apply to older people. First, isolation—a lack of social ties however measured—is a powerful risk factor for poor health. Second, social support in its many forms—emotional, actual physical assistance, and so on—has direct positive effects on health. Equally important, but less widely known, social support can buffer or reduce some of the health-related effects of aging. Finally, and perhaps most important, no single type of support is uniformly effective for all people and all situations. The effectiveness of supportive actions depends on the situation, the person, and his or her needs. Goodness of fit is essential. Unneeded or unwanted support—or the wrong kinds of support—can cause more harm than good, reducing older people's independence and self-esteem.

THE MEANING OF CONNECTEDNESS

Human beings are not meant to live solitary lives. Computer buffs would say that we are "hard-wired," genetically programmed, to develop and function by interacting with others. Talking, touching, and relating to others is essential to our well-being. These facts are not unique to children or to older men and women; they apply to all of us, from birth to death.

Like many truths about human life, this one has been discovered and rediscovered many times, and described in many ways. Thus, Rene Spitz called it hospitalism, and demonstrated a syndrome of retarded development and unresponsiveness among infants who were adequately nourished but not held, fondled, and caressed as more fortunate babies were by their parents. And consider the cases of so-called feral children, those who through some combination of disaster and neglect grew up as solitary animals, without language or human contact. Not only do they lack language and the skills that most children are taught, feral children seem to have suffered permanent developmental deficits from their lack of human contact.

Researchers at McGill University conducted a series of dramatic experiments on what they called sensory deprivation. In one such experiment, people who volunteered as experimental subjects were placed in a kind of capsule designed to eliminate or reduce as far as possible all sensory inputs. Light and sound were excluded completely, and the individual lay suspended in a bath of water kept just above body temperature. People reported that even brief exposure to this treatment produced unusual thought processes, hallucinations, and a diminished sense of both self and reality.

None of this would have surprised prisoners who have endured the special torture of prolonged solitary confinement, nor would it have surprised those who devised and imposed such penalties. Human contact is essential for normal human development and for sustained function. The needs of animals are not identical, but there is evidence that interaction with human beings affects them positively as well. We know that animals thrive under well-intentioned, loving care, including stroking, feeding, and other regular hands-on attention.

Successful agers from the MacArthur Study report that they, too, thrive as a result of important social bonds with both family and friends. Many cite friendship as the key factor in keeping them active and emotionally secure, even in advanced old age. They protect each other, share joys and concerns, and just keep each other company. Rita, seventy-nine, has a group of friends who participate in a walking group three times a week. "One watches the other, we take care of each other. It's definitely part of staying young to have friends. I miss it in rainy or snowy weather when I can't go walk. I miss my friends. If you ever have problems, you can discuss them with them and they talk to you. I wouldn't have someone else to talk to if not for them. My husband died many years ago. Most of my older friends have gone."

Stanley, eighty-two, notes that while many *human* connections keep him vital and emotionally fulfilled—his marriage, large family, church attendance, and membership in professional organizations—there are other, *nonhuman* "social" bonds that are also quite important. Gardening is one prime example in his life. "If you're involved in the garden, you're involved in living things that depend on you, and you're in a sense in a spiritual relationship with them— you do for them and they do for you. I have a dog, too, and the same can be said for her, even more so. The joy is rather like friendship, and keeps you young, because you keep concerned and happy."

A key discovery at Harvard illustrates the importance of loving support in maintaining health. The researchers bred a strain of mice lacking a gene thought to be important for learning and memory, and wanted to see what defects might occur in mice that lacked this gene. At first, the mutant mice seemed to have no abnormalities. But shortly after they gave birth, their litters died. The litters were initially healthy, however—and if the pups were taken away from their mutant mothers and raised by normal mice, they thrived. The mutant mothers simply did not take care of their pups—did not crouch over them and keep them warm, did not bring them back together when they wandered, did not help them to feed. The mutants did not harm their pups or behave aggressively toward them; they simply ignored the babies, and the lack of nurturing was fatal. Even when the mutant mothers were put in cages with normal litter-bearing females, so that the mutants could observe normal nurturing, they did not learn these behaviors or attempt to imitate them.

This finding strengthens the underlying hypothesis that the needs of human beings to relate to one another run deep, and may reflect our slowly evolved brain structure as well as the norms of human society.

CONNECTEDNESS AND SURVIVAL

Long ago it was discovered that people who committed suicide had tended to be isolated from others and withdrawn from life, a syndrome which was given the expressive French label, *anomie.* But by any name, the fact is we need continued contact with others, and the lack of such social relations is damaging. Loneliness breeds both illness and early death. And as a rule, people whose connections with others are relatively strong—through family (including marriage), friendships, and organizational memberships—live longer. And for people whose relationships to others are fewer and weaker, the risk of death is two to four times as great, irrespective of age and other factors such as race, socioeconomic status, physical health, smoking, use of alcohol, physical activity, obesity, and use of health services. The bottom line is, we do not outgrow our need for others. The life-giving effect of close social relations holds throughout the life course.

Seventy-eight-year-old Jimmy, a successful ager from the Mac-Arthur Study, found that after his wife died, nurturing friendship was the critical factor that kept him occupied and, above all else, joyful. The laughter that comes with longtime friendship imparts youth to Jimmy and to every member of his social group. "Every Thursday, I go with a couple of friends to a beautiful home with a swimming pool and we laugh our heads off. We go browsing, to Costco, Wal-Mart. They say, 'Here comes the gang.' I've been doing this for nine years, every week, since my wife passed away. And every Tuesday night I have ten or fifteen people at my house. I make pizzas. We laugh so much! We spend most of the time that way, making fun of each other. We're like a club. These are guys I grew up with, we were little kids together in East Boston. We have a ball. I instigated all this, you need one man to start it and the rest to agree. Support from friends means a lot." While Jimmy lost his best friend, a compatriot from World War II, nearly eighteen years ago, he made new, important relationships later in life. "It's all up to the person himself," he advises. "I have fifty to sixty phone numbers, and I call every one of them every holiday. If I didn't call, they'd call me and say, 'Are you okay, Jimmy?'"

SOCIAL SUPPORT: THE ESSENTIAL INGREDIENT

If close social relations are shown to help people live longer, the question is why? What is it about social relationships that extend life? And if social relationships enable people to live longer, do they also promote better, healthier lives? Do those with stronger social bonds recover more quickly or more completely from illness?

We do know this: close relationships with others involve supportive behavior, and the experience of being supported has positive effects on health.

What exactly is social support? One definition is "information leading one to believe that he or she is cared for, loved, esteemed, and a member of a network of mutual obligations." Interactions between people that communicate such information protect them from many of the damaging health effects of stressful life events. And that protection is quite wide-ranging, including a lower risk of arthritis, tuberculosis, depression, and alcoholism. People who say that they receive strong social support also require less pain medication after surgery, recover more quickly, and follow medical regimens more faithfully. These are not "all or none" findings; social support is not magic, but in all these stressful situations, people who had more support did better than those who had less or none at all.

The next critical questions, of course, are, "What does supportive behavior consist of?" and "Why is support supportive?" That is, what are the mechanisms by which social support protects people against stress and enhances their health? And how do the benefits of social support apply to older men and women?

What Does Social Support Consist Of?

Social support carries many meanings, including such factors as information, trust, care, love, esteem, network membership, and mutual obligation. In general, two kinds of support are important for successful aging: so-called socioemotional support and instrumental support. Socioemotional support includes direct expressions of affection, liking, love, esteem, and respect. Instrumental support involves hands-on assistance in some activity, such as care when ill, help with household chores, providing transportation, loans or gifts of money, and the like. The first kind of support—emotional—is extremely important for successful aging. The second is sometimes less so, as we'll discuss further.

Why Is Support Supportive?

There are four important ways in which support may promote health. First, it is possible that support helps one to obtain better or prompter medical care. Second, some kinds of social support may actually come in the form of medical care. Third, social support may increase conformity to group norms that are health promotive, such as starting walking groups or not smoking. And fourth, supportive behaviors may have biological effects that directly increase one's resistance to disease. All four mechanisms are plausible. For instance, encouragement and reassurance can help a person to overcome fearfulness about seeking medical treatment, and information can help in the choice of physician or medical facility. Direct assistance during illness can take the form of medical or nursing care—for example, administering medication on schedule or helping a bedridden person to change positions and thus prevent bedsores. And so on.

Unfortunately, in some cases well-intentioned but inappropriate supportive behavior can also work against such positive outcomes.

Naive reassurance about some symptom—"My grandfather had a lump like that and he lived to be 103"—can postpone medical diagnosis and lovingly administered home remedies sometimes do more harm than good. The power of group norms can help people keep to diet and exercise regimens, but the power of the group has also led many a teenager to begin a lifelong habit of cigarette smoking. In short, for social support to have positive effects, it must be appropriate as well as well-intentioned.

There is a good deal of evidence that social support provides some chronic and continuing protective effect. For instance, in general, married people live longer than unmarried people, and members of church and secular organizations live longer than people without such group affiliations. And older women who say they have little opportunity to talk to others about their problems tend to have higher blood pressure than those who are better connected. But what about the fact that social support seems also to protect against *acute* or immediate health threats? How might this be explained?

Consider a study of women about to give birth in a Guatemalan hospital, which usually requires women to be alone during labor. The women were randomly assigned to an experimental or a control group. Those in the control group followed the usual hospital procedures—and were alone until delivery. The others were accompanied by a woman, otherwise untrained, who was instructed to provide physical contact, conversation, and friendly companionship during labor and delivery. The women who received emotional support had shorter labors, fewer complications, and were more wakeful and attentive to their infants than the women who gave birth alone.

SUPPORT IN OLD AGE

Most research on social support has been done without attention to age, and yet the need for support and the ability to provide it to others surely changes as we move through the life course. However, the common view of old age as a prolonged period of demanding support from an ever-diminishing number of overworked providers is wrong. The truth about older men and women is much more encouraging.

The Convoy of Social Support

There is surprising stability in the size of support networks throughout the life course. Critical factors in successful aging are how many supportive people one has in one's "inner circle," and what kind of support they give.

Imagine yourself a respondent to a survey of social relationships among older people. The interviewer begins by handing you a diagram that looks like a target for teaching marksmanship. It consists of three concentric circles, unlabeled, and a bull's-eye that contains a single word, "you." The interviewer explains that the diagram is intended to help you think of the people who are important in your life right now, and the three concentric circles represent different degrees of importance. People in the innermost circle are those "to whom you feel so close that it is hard to imagine life without them. If there are any people like that in your life, let's begin with them." People in the next circles are also important to you and your relationships with them are close, but less so. The mapping process continues until the members of your personal network have been identified by initials or nicknames and located on the diagram. The interview then shifts to questions about each relationship, especially the nature and extent of support given and received.

Typical Support Circles

What have we learned? There are three important findings. First, most people of all ages (who live in private households rather than retirement or nursing homes) report a considerable number of close relationships with others. Some people do suffer from isolation and loneliness but, on the average, people of all ages report that their personal networks include eight to eleven members. Second, network size is quite stable across the life course. Age is not irrelevant to network size; people between thirty-five and fifty years of age tend to have larger networks than those who are either younger or older. But the differences are not large, and the overall finding is one of stability. Third, people's support networks often change over the course of a lifetime. There are losses—mainly through death, changes in residence, and retirement—but there are also replacements, so that the losses do not necessarily produce a net reduction in network size.

We like the term "convoy of social support" to describe the pattern of supportive relationships with which an individual moves through life. A convoy is a dynamic entity; the ships that make it up are in motion, en route to a destination. They are protected by being part of the convoy, but each also provides a degree of protection to the others. The metaphor of the convoy seems to fit the personal networks of stability and change on which we depend for support as we move through the life course.

Several successful agers describe their "convoys" as a vital means of escaping the potential loneliness and isolation of old age. And many say the more diverse the group, the better—young, old, relatives, friends, and so on. Jean, seventy-nine, doesn't think of herself as older and tries to spend time with people who feel the same way. "Having a wide network of people, friends, is a good thing. The people I see are very active—going to concerts and so on. I have friends of all ages, just had lunch with a woman half my age. I do very well alone, but you can only read so many books. Since I live alone, it's important. I am lucky in many ways, I have several good friends, all determined and all doing interesting things. The circle of friends is important."

For men and women whose spouse is still alive, the spouse may provide a vast amount of emotional and social support. Gesamino, a MacArthur Study successful ager, firmly believes that his romantic and sexual relationship with his wife is a major factor in his retained youth: "I tell her I love her, I hug her and kiss her. I take her for dinners, dancing. Thirty-five years. If a man is married he should love his wife, make her happy and your life and health will be better because of it. I am seventy-nine, my wife is sixty-one. We both enjoy sex between the two of us, and we go out and have a good time. You've got to treat your wife like a queen—and she treats me the same way."

Reciprocity Over the Life Course

When older people are asked with whom they share six main kinds of support—confiding, reassuring, providing sick care, expressing respect or affection, talking about health or about problems—they often name the people from their "inner circle," especially the spouse, adult children, and other immediate family members. Close friends are sometimes mentioned in the inner circle, but are more likely to be located in the middle or outer circle, along with neighbors, coworkers, and relatives outside the immediate family.

These patterns of support change quite little over the lifetime—less than most people would expect. All six of the main forms of support are both provided and received by people in every age group. Moreover, the overall amount of support that people report receiving does not increase significantly with age. There are age-related changes, however, in the pattern of support; the need for sick care, for example, is greater in the oldest age group. There is an age-related change also in reciprocity, the balance between support receiving and support providing. The amount of support that people report providing to others goes down with age; younger people report providing more support to others than older people do.

The amount of reported reciprocity is greatest between spouses, less with other family members including children, and still less with friends. It is a sad irony that the death of a spouse means the loss of the survivor's primary source of social support at a moment when the fact of bereavement greatly heightens the need for support. However, some successful agers from the MacArthur Study say that *giving* emotional and other support is more important than receiving it, and that the process of giving can distract one from the pain of major emotional losses, such as a spouse's death. After Anne, eighty-seven, lost her husband, she simply refused to let herself wallow in grief. She cleans, cooks, shops, drives, and does just about every imaginable task for herself. And most important, she cares for her disabled grandson, and finds that "this emotional giving fills the void lost when my husband died. I think keeping busy, not dwelling on the past, helps. You can't let your hands hang by your sides."

SOCIAL SUPPORT AND HEALTH

People who have a great deal of social support are healthier, on average, than people who lack such support. That assertion, after more than two decades of research, is no longer debated. But the ever-recurring question of *why* is again before us. What is it about social support that is health promotive? What are the psychobiological mechanisms by which the health-giving properties of social support, whatever they are, have their effects? Answers to these questions are not only important for scientific understanding; they are crucial for effective action.

The more older people participate in social relationships, the better their overall health. A variety of different venues of social contact and support promote successful aging. These include telephone conversations with friends, relatives, or neighbors; visits with friends, relatives, or neighbors; participation in religious groups; and attendance at meetings of organizations. Among men and women sixty years of age or more, all these interactions predicted "robust aging," an index of overall well-being that includes involvement in productive activity, emotional and mental status, and functional level. The two strongest predictors of well-being are frequency of visits with friends and frequency of attending meetings of organizations. Interestingly, the more meaningful the contribution in a given activity, the greater its impact on health. For instance, those who actually attend religious meetings do better than those who simply say they are religious. Active participation does a person more good than mere attendance.

One MacArthur Study successful ager tells us that her faith in God is the supreme factor in allowing her to survive into late life. Mary, eighty, has endured the deaths of three brothers, her husband, and more recently, her daughter-in-law. But her religious activities and belief have buffered the emotional blow of these enormous losses. "I always have a lot of faith. The good Lord has always given me the strength to go on. I was raised to believe and pray when I have problems. I go to Mass every Sunday, and we have other special days when we go to Mass. I'm a eucharistic minister. God makes me do things to feel better—I serve people and God. I go to buildings to give Communion to people who can't get out." Mary's religious activity leads to both the giving and receiving of support. While her congregation and faith give her strength, they also provide a context in which she can help others. And this, in turn, helps distract her from the pain she has faced throughout her lifetime.

BIOCHEMICAL CHANGES CAUSED BY EMOTIONAL SUPPORT

People's stories of the value of the emotional support they give and receive are important—but they are also subjective. The MacArthur Studies looked beyond people's feelings and beliefs, and searched for hard facts—that is, physiological effects of support. We found clear evidence that social support can have important physiological as well as psychological effects. The effects differ, however, depending on the type of support provided and the outcome under study. And the effects of support are different for men than for women.

The MacArthur Study looked at men and women seventy to seventy-nine years of age who were relatively high-functioning at the time of the initial interview; that is, their physical and cognitive performance put them in the upper one-third of their age group. Even within this generally high-functioning group, those who reported greater emotional support from their network members scored higher in physical performance. *Men* who reported high social support also had significantly lower levels of three physiological measures of stress—epinephrine, norepinephrine, and cortisol—known colloquially as the "stress hormones." This buffering of stress hormones was not apparent for women, however.

GOODNESS OF FIT

Not all supportive actions have their intended effects. Unwanted or unneeded support can backfire. Just as when one provides too much assistance to a child, that young person can fail to develop independent skills and self-esteem, so too it is possible to provide "too much of a good thing" to elders. In contrast to the generally positive relationship between emotional support and physical performance, the kinds of direct assistance that are called "instrumental support" (e.g., helping someone with a task) are associated with *lower* physical performance in older people. Even if that assistance was given with the best intentions, providing more assistance than people really need can reduce their belief in themselves, as well as their ability to function. The current slogan of "use it or lose it" applies not only to exercise and athletic ability, but to basic physical and cognitive functions as well.

Giving direct assistance in excess of what people need or perhaps want is a frequent, well-meant, but mistaken form of support. Most parents have had the experience of teaching a young child to ride a two-wheeled bicycle. At some point in the learning process, the parent is trotting along with one hand on the bicycle seat to steady the young rider. But as the rider gets up to speed and acquires a sense of balance, the parental hand is no longer wanted and continued assistance is strongly discouraged. "Let go! I'm okay! I can do it myself!"

Older men and women, given more help than they need, may be less assertive in discouraging it. But the unneeded assistance, even if it is welcomed, has its price. Older people who are prevented from helping themselves tend toward a state of "learned helplessness."

In the MacArthur Study, people who were relatively low in their sense of self-efficacy tended to decline in their ability to function during the two and a half years between the initial and subsequent assessments. Specifically, they were more likely to report that they needed help with bathing, dressing, eating, using the toilet, walking across a small room, or moving from bed to chair. Strong belief in one's abilities, on the other hand, protects people against such functional decline, and the protective effect is strongest among people who actually showed some loss in objective performance tests (tapping their feet, getting up from a chair, speed walking, etc.).

And so we argue that not all intended support is a good thing. To maximize successful aging, one must assess the needs of the individual, the situation, and the type and amount of support needed. And clearly, we must remember that support acts as a safety net.

Anna, eighty-one, is another MacArthur successful ager. Her emotional safety net consists of her husband, twin sister, and three other siblings. Hers is a dedicated family—the net is always at hand. "We're very close. That has a lot to do with staying young, because you always have someone there for you. We do things together. We go to bingo. Every Wednesday we go to a different house for cards. My twin and I used to do oil painting at the senior center—we plan to get back to that. There's always someone to talk to." Whether a problem arises or not, the possibility of support is present—the words assumed, but often unsaid. Just knowing the net is there confers adequate protection. It is not necessary to fall.

CHAPTER ELEVEN

PRODUCTIVITY IN OLD AGE

How dull it is to pause, to make an end,
To rust unburnished, not to shine in use!
As though to breathe were life!
—TENNYSON

POETRY AND PROSE

The lines above are from "Ulysses," one of Tennyson's greatest poems. It begins where Homer left off. Ulysses, the great adventurer, has long since found his way back to Ithaca, his island kingdom, and to Penelope, his beloved and resourceful wife. He now speaks as an old man, who is discovering that the home and even the love that he yearned for in his wanderings are not enough. An old age of idleness is becoming a burden rather than a gift; he yearns to "shine in use."

Freud's assertion that love and work are the essentials of human life speaks the same truth without the poetry. Our concept of successful aging includes these ideas and builds on them. We defined successful aging as including three main components: low probability of disease and disability, high mental and physical function, and active engagement with life. For active engagement with life, the key elements are two: close personal relationships with family and friends, and continued involvement in productive activities. Freud's translation says it in two syllables: love, work. We turn now to the nature and meaning of work in old age.

THE AMBIVALENCE OF SOCIETY

Our society is of two minds about productivity in old age. On the one hand, jobs—especially good jobs—seem scarce, and some younger people resent the fact that their elders are taking up wanted positions. True, our official unemployment rate, currently under 5 percent, is the envy of most other countries. Nevertheless, millions of people are looking for work; millions who are working less than full-time want more work; and unnumbered others go to their jobs in fear of unemployment. The sight of older people holding tenaciously to jobs coveted by younger men and women is not conducive to intergenerational harmony. It is now illegal to compel workers to retire because of age alone, but that fact adds force to the argument that greedy old workers should make way for needy young workers.

On the other hand, we are told that lack of productivity among older men and women is a major national problem. Congressional deliberations each year about the national budget always include warnings from one or another senator and representative that the nation "cannot afford" its increasing proportion of older men and women. The underlying issue in the debate is the productivity of older men and women as compared to their consumption of goods and services, especially medical care. To add a bit of arithmetic to the assertion that the survival of the elderly imposes an unbearable economic burden on the rest of society, speakers point to the "dependency ratio," a simple comparison between the number of people in paid employment and the number not so employed.

If one of us (RLK), as a citizen now venturing cheerfully into his eightieth year, wanted to satisfy both sides of this argument—make way for youth but don't add to its economic burden—he would be perplexed. Should he try to reenter the labor market and pay his way or stay out of it and leave his hypothetical job to a younger man or woman? Such is the literal or figurative dilemma facing many an older person in our society. Put that way, the question allows no satisfactory answer: in both cases, the older person represents burden, not asset.

FACT AND FICTION

Fortunately, the picture is not as it appears on the surface. The "dependency ratio" gives a false image of what older people are already contributing and gives no hint of their potential for making greater contributions. The confusion begins by defining all paid employment as productive and all unpaid activity as unproductive. That error is built into our national statistics, which define the Gross Domestic Product (GDP) in terms of paid activities and exclude all unpaid ones. A woman or man who cares for a disabled friend or family member without pay is not included in the official count of employed and productive people. Were that same person to be providing the same care for pay, the activity would suddenly become productive. A sales clerk in a hospital gift shop is considered productive if she or he is paid, but unproductive if she or he is a volunteer. Rae André, who was particularly concerned with the official underestimation of women's work, suggested that a pair of friendly neighbors could clean each other's houses instead of each their own. Each could pay the other for doing so and both would suddenly be recognized as productive. More to the pragmatic point, both would become eligible for unemployment benefits and Social Security entitlements.

The MacArthur Studies in Successful Aging began with a different and more realistic definition of productive behavior: any activity, paid or unpaid, that generates goods or services of economic value is productive. This definition lets us discover what older people really contribute. Several studies have now taken this approach, and together they tell a very different and encouraging story about productive activity among older men and women.

WHAT OLDER PEOPLE REALLY DO

There are three short answers to the question of what older people really do: 1) most older men and women do some productive work; 2) all in all, the amount of such work is substantial; and 3) much of it continues throughout life. Of course, these general statements tell only part of the story; individual differences among older people are very large. But the generalizations deserve some attention.

Most older people make productive contributions of some kind, more in the form of informal help giving and unpaid volunteer work than paid employment. Among people fifty-five years of age and older, more than nine out of ten do housework; eight out of ten do home maintenance or improvement; seven out of ten provide help of various kinds to friends and relatives; and more than three out of ten work as volunteers in churches, hospitals, and other organizations. Almost as many older people work for pay as volunteer, about three out of ten. Taking all these activities together, we find that almost all older people living in private households engage in some forms of productive activity; only 2 percent report none whatsoever.

We discussed productivity and work with some of the Mac-Arthur Study successful agers. Many are actively engaged in various types of unpaid and paid work, and they often attributed their ongoing vitality to their occupations. They also spoke of the meaning of being *needed*—and how that keeps them going. Eighty-three-year-old Rose is active in several political organizations, where she volunteers to do mailings and other odd tasks. She also runs an animal shelter in her home, bringing abandoned animals into her big old house by the drove. "Every day is a busy day. I get a lot of happiness knowing these little critters have a home. I'm just not ready to lay down and die. I think the Good Lord is going to have to grab me by my coattails and drag me."

John, age eighty, volunteers in his church and also tends to an aging neighbor: "I watch over him like a mother hen and he shows his appreciation. It makes me feel good to know I'm helping him." And eighty-year-old Carmen works three days a week teaching barbering. "It keeps me active, keeps my mind sharp, keeps me alert, keeps my blood moving," he says. Beatrice, eighty-one, who recently chaired a luncheon honoring centenarians in her community, sums it up nicely when she says, "I hope to die with my boots on. I've got to be doing something. I've got a wish list of things I want done in the community. An intergenerational program at one of the facilities I work in. A work program where older people can earn money so they'll feel worth something. I fill my time." All of these successful agers have learned the value of active engagement in life, doing for others, challenging the mind or the body on a regular basis—in sum, keeping the wheels turning year in and year out, so they don't get rusty or stop altogether.

The amount of work done by older men and women is substantial. Not only do almost all older people work, they work many hours. Among those fifty-five years of age or older, more than four out of ten report at least 1,500 hours of productive activity during the year. About as many report working 500 to 1,499 hours, and fewer than two out of ten are in the lightest work category—1 to 499 hours during the year. The curriculum vitae of Frank Stanton, who retired as vice chairman of CBS in 1973 after serving as president there from 1946 until 1971, says a great deal more than any statistic can reveal. After retiring from his longtime position at CBS, he began serving actively on the boards of major companies from New York Life to the International Herald Tribune. Today, at the age of eighty-nine, he describes himself as "slowed down" (without any intended humor), while maintaining an active office, serving as board director of two major mutual funds, board director of Sony Music, overseer of Harvard College, and playing a meaningful role in a dense list of activities that many people a third his age couldn't manage. When asked for an explanation of his tremendous productivity in late life, he refuses to boast—but does offer serious advice to others in his peer group about how to remain productive in old age. "Don't do it with your left hand," he stresses. "Throw yourself in, give it all you've got. Too many people do it halfway. Find voluntary work if you don't have a paid option." A certain major athletic shoe company motto comes to mind: "Just Do It." Frank Stanton certainly does.

It is true that most people tend to reduce their total amount of productive activity as they get older, but the pattern of reduction is different for each activity. Hours spent at different kinds of work peak and decline at different stages of the life course. For instance, child care peaks early, when parents are in the twenty-five- to thirty-four-year age range and children are young. Hours of child care decline sharply after age forty-five, but they go up slightly among people aged sixty-five to seventy-four, reminding us that grandparents do a significant amount of that work. Hours of paid work peak early and are sustained until the conventional age of retirement; they drop sharply after age sixty-five. Hours of volunteer work peak somewhat later, but are much more stable. Informal help to friends and relatives peaks still later, in the fifty-five- to sixty-four-year age range, as people respond to the increasing needs of those they are close to. Providing such help, both for chronic and acute problems, continues to age seventy-five and beyond. On average, men and women in this oldest group spend as much time helping friends and relatives as do people half their age.

Clearly, after age fifty-five, unpaid work is the main form of productive activity for both men and women, and it continues into very old age. The bias of counting only paid work as productive now becomes clear: it creates a gross underestimation of productive work at all ages, greater underestimation for women than for men, and a proportionately greater underestimation for people in middle and old age than for those in young adulthood.

WHAT IT TAKES TO BE PRODUCTIVE

The MacArthur Studies on Successful Aging tell us a great deal about what it takes to be productive in old age. Three factors stand out as promoting later-life productivity: health and overall ability to function; participation in friendship and other social relations; and personal characteristics, such as being better educated and believing in one's ability to handle what life has to offer.

Mental and Physical Function

It makes sense that the better one can function mentally and physically, the more likely one is to work, both for pay and as a volunteer. Older men and women who score high in mental and physical function are three times as likely as low-functioning seniors to be doing paid work and more than twice as likely to be working as volunteers. High mental and physical function probably both facilitates productive work and strengthens the need and wish to be active. And not surprisingly, people who rate their own health positively, and who report few chronic conditions or none at all, are more likely to be productive than those whose health is more problematical.

People who report problems with vision or difficulty in meeting the daily requirements of personal care are, as would be expected, less likely than others to engage in productive activity. Hospitalizations and acute health problems like stroke often lead, as we would expect, to reduced productivity.

However, some people remain productive *in spite of* functional limitations and chronic diseases, and no one should feel that such limitations make it impossible to be productive. Take the case of Phyllis, eighty, who continues to work as an actress despite three heart attacks, major heart surgery, colon cancer, and a serious fall that led to lung failure and more heart problems. Phyllis continues to perform as regularly as possible, auditioning for the fewer and fewer roles available to older women. She is on stage two to three months a year, and when she is not in a show, she fills her time with volunteer work in the theater world, serving at the box office, doing mailings, and so on. And she is an avid theatergoer as well. The secret to her ability to move forward and remain productive in the face of serious physical problems is quite simple: "Keep your interest in outer things, not inner ones. Keep busy. And always maintain more interests than there's time for."

Friendship and Social Relations

Continuing relations with others have long been recognized as important for well-being. Although people differ in their need for interaction with others, human beings are not programmed for prolonged isolation. Older men and women who report frequent visits with friends and attendance at meetings are more likely to be engaged in productive activities. People who are not married and who live alone more often showed reductions in such activities. This makes sense. After all, being part of an active network of other human beings increases the opportunity and the motivation for productivity of many kinds.

Enduring Personal Characteristics

People who have had more years of education are more likely to be productive in old age. So many studies have found this to be true, that the finding itself is beyond question; however, the mechanisms by which education leads to late-life productivity have yet to be fully discovered. At least two explanations for the education-productivity relationship are plausible and both may be at work.

One possibility is that education affects productivity because of its influence on socioeconomic status. Education determines access to occupations and occupations determine income. Income in turn shapes the life course in many ways—place of residence, social contacts, and leisure activities among them. People who have acquired the experience and skills that higher-level income and occupation confer are likely to enter old age in better health and with greater knowledge of opportunities for volunteerism.

Another possibility is that education brings about changes in the individual man or woman that are lifelong and that express themselves in many ways, of which late-life productivity is only one.

Willingness to improve one's education as one ages may also promote later-life productivity. Ron worked for thirty-two years as a nuclear engineer. He started to witness the ups and downs of his industry and began to worry about his financial future. At the age of fifty-seven, Ron decided he must learn another trade in order to have something to fall back on as he grew older. He selected his brother-in-law's profession, accounting, and started to take courses in the subject. A tuition refund program at his old job helped fund the schooling—he persuaded his bosses that every manager should have some accounting skills. Later, he took and passed the CPA exam and got his license to practice. Today, at sixty-nine, he works at least a thirty-five-hour week (and more during tax season). He finds that the income helps (though with Social Security limits up to age seventy, this has been minor), but equally important, he says that the work "keeps the brain from atrophying. I didn't want to sit in the house. I don't play golf. There are only so many books you can read. As an engineer I was trained to look toward the completion of a program, a goal. I needed to go *toward* something."

In addition to education, the second personal characteristic that predicts productive activity among older men and women is "self-efficacy," which refers to a person's belief in his or her ability to deal with different situations in a competent manner. In other words, when we are confronted with a challenge or an opportunity to take action, we ask ourselves the silent question "Am I capable of doing this successfully?" Our level of self-efficacy determines the answer, and therefore the probability that the action will be attempted, the opportunity taken.

In the MacArthur Studies, a sense of mastery—that is, a person's belief in his or her ability to influence events and control their outcomes—also proved to be important in promoting productive behavior. During a period of less than three years, people whose sense of mastery increased also increased their amount of productive activity; those whose sense of mastery decreased also reduced their involvement in productive activities.

Interestingly, we know that the opposite is true, as well: having a passive approach to life, that is, a feeling that one is unable to take actions that shape one's own life, promotes *lack* of productivity.

Belief in one's abilities and the sense that one can, to some extent, control one's destiny tends to persist as we age. Many experiments have proved, however, that a positive sense of self can be created in those who lack it. Self-efficacy *can* be increased. For instance, people with a fear of flying can become relatively comfortable with airline travel. People with a very low ability to tolerate pain can learn to deal with it realistically. Cardiac patients who had no confidence in their ability to attain certain levels of physical activity have regained a sense of their ability to improve their lives, and have boosted both their treadmill performance and, more important, their involvement in life activities.

What does it take to make the shift to greater self-reliance, belief in oneself, and healthy, active behavior? It takes three important factors: 1) an opportunity to undertake a specific action that challenges one's sense of self-sufficiency *without* overwhelming it; 2) the presence of supportive and reassuring others; and 3) the experience of succeeding at something, with confirming feedback from others. A sense of power and self-worth is a sort of built-in self-fulfilling prophecy; confidence in one's ability to do a thing successfully increases both the likelihood of undertaking it and the probability of success. It is almost certain that increasing older people's sense of self-esteem and competence will increase their productive behavior. Nor is that all: bringing less active older people into productive activities, with appropriate support and encouraging feedback, might also enhance their sense of self-efficacy and thus initiate a "virtuous cycle" to replace a "vicious" one.

WHAT DO OLDER PEOPLE WANT?

This is a simple question to ask, but a difficult one to answer. Of course, surveys can ask older men and women how they would prefer to spend their time, but few surveys have done so. Even those surveys that have asked older people what they do—or want to do—are subject to biased answers. Certainly it is less socially desirable to say that you would prefer to spend your time watching television and drinking beer than to say that you would like to work as a volunteer in a shelter for the homeless. Furthermore, when older men or women tell you realistically what they would like to be doing, they are necessarily speaking on the basis of their experience of the world as it is. The possibilities that they see may therefore be very limited, and may greatly understate their potential. With these limitations in mind, then, let us consider what is known about the attitudes and values of older men and women with respect to productive activities, paid and unpaid.

"OUGHTS" AND "SHOULDS": THE QUESTION OF VALUES

We will begin with values, those inner voices that tell us what we ourselves and others ought to do and not do. *"After a life of work and service, retirement and leisure are well deserved." "Over a lifetime, there should be time to grow, time to work, and finally time to rest."* Among people sixty years of age and over, more than nine out of ten agree with those statements, and most of them agree strongly.

Clearly, older people do not feel guilty or disapproving about increased rest and leisure in old age. On the other hand, they agree with the following statement almost as strongly as those quoted above: "*A person should continue to work as long as he or she is able.*" Apparently they think of a leisure-saturated, passive retirement as something that is justified only by the lack of ability for work. However, about as many older people agree with the following statement as disagree with it: "*Older people should step down from their responsibilities and let younger people take their place.*" These value preferences are driven by still deeper convictions. "*Life is not worth living if one cannot contribute to the well-being of others.*" "*Older people who no longer work should contribute through community service.*" About eight out of ten older people agree with both these statements, more strongly with the first than the second. With regard to these values, the frequent gulf between old and young does not appear.

With respect to work, what people want for themselves is generally consistent with what they advocate for others. People who are working for pay want to keep on doing so. Older surveys included the question of whether people would want to keep on working even if they had no economic need to do so. In 1953, when that question was first asked of a national sample, almost 75 percent of all employed men said they would want to work, irrespective of financial need. The percentage was less for women, but the majority of them gave the same response. The percentage also decreased with age, but it remained the majority response among men in the fifty-five- to sixty-four-year age range. It reduced somewhat for all age groups during the 1960s, perhaps suggesting some erosion of the work ethic, but was stable during the 1970s. Comparable data are not available for recent years.

The reasons people gave for wanting to continue working, aside from the need for money, mainly involve social relations and the use of time. Working relationships often become friendships and the routines of work give a kind of organization to the day that people say they would miss. Only one person in ten gives "enjoying the work itself" as a reason to continue working, and further questioning makes it clear that, for most people, wanting to continue working does not mean wanting to continue at the same job or with the same hours. Some people want more hours of work and some less, but the wish for less work is the more common response in later life; among employed people between the ages of fifty-five and seventy, at least twice as many want less work as those who want more.

People are skeptical, however, about the likelihood of getting the kind of paid work that they want and the amount of it that they want. And their experience confirms their skepticism. Among people fifty to seventy years of age, about four out of ten wanted less work, but three years later only one in ten had gotten it. People who wanted *more* work (about 2 out of 10) were even less likely to get their wish. The gap between work wanted and work offered explains in part people's decision to retire. They see the choice as either continuing to work without a change in job content or hours—or quitting entirely—and they choose to quit.

WORDS AND DEEDS

People, old and young, believe in the value of a productive life. They rate the benefits of regular paid work highly. On a scale ranging from a low of one to a high of four, a national sample of adults rated paid work 3.4 in benefit to themselves and 3.3 in benefit to others. These high ratings do not depend entirely on work as a source of income, however. People rate *unpaid* work—child care, volunteer work, and informal help to others—as highly as paid work in terms of benefit to themselves. And they rate unpaid work even higher than paid work in terms of its benefit to others. Volunteer work, for example, is rated 3.55 in benefit to others, second only to child care.

Jean, eighty-seven, works as a volunteer for three half-days each week. She took up the job in her late seventies. Most of her work is in the area of legal services, where she serves as a file clerk and librarian. She had spent many years of time and money in voluntary pursuits that brought her little satisfaction. Then she switched to "where it counted," the legal world. "It's irritating but satisfying," she admits. "I keep track of everything, they don't have anybody else to do it. I know that without me they'd have to hire someone. The lawyers are young and it's a dedicated environment—I'm proud that I can contribute. People expect older people to be tottering into a nursing home. But I never conform to what people expect, I'm feisty to begin with. I'm just curious all the time, natively curious. As a kid, I turned stones over to see the beetles underneath. And I ate the beetles, maybe because my cat ate them. Figuratively, I'm still eating beetles."

Feisty volunteers like Jean are relatively rare. Fewer than one-third of all older men and women work as volunteers and those who do spend, on average, fewer than two hours a week on the job. Civic, religious, medical, educational, and environmental organizations, meanwhile, are eager for volunteers. Earlier in their history, many of these organizations depended mainly on women, often highly educated and competent women who were not employed at paid work. In this era of two-worker families, these voluntary organizations find that their main source of talent and energy has moved from the unpaid to the paid labor force.

The leaders of voluntary organizations have not yet learned, however, how to reach out to the active and able elderly. Employers are only beginning to show the kind of flexibility that lets older people continue or resume paid work. Older men and women themselves, while many of them recognize and enjoy their continued vitality, have yet to realize the full range of its use. And research, which has already discovered many of the factors that enable productivity in old age, has yet to discover how best to increase the numbers of older people who age successfully in that important way.

In short, and not for the first time in human affairs, our deeds lag behind our words. How best to close that gap is a challenge to individuals and to organizations. Our own proposals are the subject of the final chapter in this book.

CHAPTER TWELVE

PRESCRIPTIONS FOR AN AGING SOCIETY

AGING: THEN AND NOW

Not too many years ago, on the walls of many American homes hung a reproduction of a particular painting. I (RLK) saw it first as a child; I remember it hanging in the bedroom of my favorite aunt. The picture puzzled me: I found it somber and even a little frightening, as much because of its lack of color as its subject. The artist had called it *Arrangement in Grey and Black No. 1,* but most people called it *Whistler's Mother,* and it was with that name that it had become famous. It is a portrait of an older woman, exactly how old is not clear. She sits in profile, unmoving, a lace cap on her head, and perhaps a dark blanket or robe across her knees. Her expression is hard to interpret: severity? tranquillity? resignation?

The artist, James Abbott McNeill Whistler, painted the picture when he was thirty-seven years old and his mother was sixty-seven. The appeal of the portrait is not easy to understand here at the end of the twentieth century, but perhaps it symbolized the nineteenth-century view of proper old age: sit quietly and wait for the end. In any case, it reminds us of how greatly the realities of aging and, more slowly, the perceptions of older people have changed during the past 100 years.

In this chapter we first review those changes, many of which have been discussed in detail earlier in this book. We then consider the attitudes of others toward older people, the expectations people have about the behavior of older men and women, and the opportunities and supportive services that are available to them.

In the preceding chapters of this book, we have concentrated on individuals—their experience of aging, the things that reduce their risk of disease and disability, maintain their physical and cognitive function, and their engagement with life. The emphasis has been on what people themselves can do to age successfully. Now we shift gears, and think at the level of community facilities and national policy. Decisions and resources at community, state, and national levels affect the probability that each of us can age successfully. Finally, we consider the policy changes that might make successful aging the majority experience and imagine the contributions that a majority of successful agers could make to the larger society.

CHANGES IN LIFE EXPECTANCY

In the long course of human history there are no instances of terrestrial immortality—the fact of human mortality is unchanging. What has changed, and changed greatly, is life expectancy, the number of years that newborn infants can be expected to live, on average. For most of recorded human history and the 100,000 years of human prehistory, life expectancy was very low. Birth rates were high, but so was infant mortality, early death from infectious disease, and deadly encounters with men and beasts. Life expectancy at the time of the Roman empire was about twenty-eight years. Roman civilization, remarkably advanced in so many domains, was not able to prevent high rates of death in infancy or the lifelong threat of deadly infectious disease. From the birth of Christ to 1900, each year of history saw an average gain of three days in life expectancy. Each year since 1900, however, has seen a gain of 110 days in average life expectancy.

Some authorities warn us, and with reason, about the development of new drug-resistant strains of viruses and bacteria and the emergence of new diseases. The spread of AIDS confronts us with the magnitude of such threats. Nevertheless, as discussed in the introduction to this book, the recent and continuing gains in life expectancy have come mainly from reduced death rates in the adult years, especially in middle and old age. Dramatic improvements in surgery, development of new diagnostic equipment and procedures, and the creation of new drugs for the management of chronic diseases are largely responsible for these gains. Reduction in the proportion of men who are cigarette smokers will contribute as well. Other behavioral changes that would increase life expectancy—changes in diet, increased exercise, and reduced cigarette use by women, for example—are potential sources of further gain rather than explanations for gains already observable.

SOME IMPLICATIONS OF LONGER LIFE

The effects of these changes in the length of life are many and are still unfolding. Some are already beyond question; the countries that have experienced the greatest increases in life expectancy have also had marked reductions in birth rates. It is as if people decide to have fewer children when they are assured that their children will survive. The technological advancement and general prosperity that contribute to extended life also make the means of contraception widely available.

The increased presence of older men and women is beyond debate. But while these facts are certain, at least three related questions are hotly contested: Does longer life mean more years of health or of illness? What is the limit to human life? And are increased numbers of older men and women an asset or a burden to the larger society? We discuss the answer to the first question in chapter 1, myth #1—To be old is to be sick. The limits to human life, if any, are discussed in the Introduction. We turn now to the third question.

OLDER MEN AND WOMEN: ASSET OR BURDEN?

Policy decisions affecting older people reflect the perceptions and attitudes of policy makers and legislators at levels from local to national, executives of organizations, and decision makers throughout the nation. Their perception of older people as either an asset or a burden to the rest of society involves three additional questions: how many older people are there? what do they take? and what do they give?

On the first of these questions, there is near unanimity. Both the numbers of older people and their proportion of the total population are increasing and will continue to do so for decades to come. Members of the baby boom generation, those infants born in the early years after World War II, are now moving into middle age and altering the age composition of the population as they themselves age.

There is widespread agreement that these increasing numbers give greater importance to policy decisions that affect the elderly— especially decisions regarding Social Security, medical care, and other entitlements. This is where the agreement stops, however. Policy makers disagree about the obligations of government and the responsibilities of individuals, about the contributions of older people and about their demands. They disagree, in short, on whether older men and women are an asset or a burden to society as a whole.

What They Get: Entitlements and Expectations

The entitlements of older people are of two main kinds—pensions (primarily Social Security) and health care (primarily Medicare). Both are extremely important to the well-being of the elderly, and both contribute to the stereotype of older men and women as affluent in income and extravagant in the use of medical services. The facts, as always, are more complex than the stereotypes.

The dollar income of elderly households (defined as those whose members are sixty years of age or over) is less than two-thirds (64 percent) that of younger households. However, the households of older people are usually smaller than those of younger; if we take that fact into account, the money incomes of elderly and younger households are about equal. If we make a further adjustment to take nonmonetary income into account, the income advantage shifts to the elderly, mainly because of their use of Medicare and their equity in home ownership. The individual situations of older people vary greatly, however; in 1992 only 15 percent of older men and women had any financial assets in addition to Social Security and home equity, and almost as many (12 percent) were living below the poverty line.

The stereotype of the elderly as extravagant users of medical care and as the primary cause of increasing medical costs is another mix of fact and fiction. Certainly older people take more medicines, spend more days in hospitals, and see doctors more frequently than young people do. About 12 percent of the population are over age sixty-five, but that group uses 25 percent of all prescribed medications, 40 percent of bed-days in hospitals, and 33 percent of all health expenditures. Those are significant differences, but they do not tell us that the elderly are the majority consumers of health care.

As people grow older, they do need more help in activities of daily living—bathing, dressing, eating, and moving from bed to chair. At age sixty-five, 10 to 20 percent of a person's remaining years are likely to be spent dependent in one or more of these ways. By age eighty-five, about half of people's remaining time is likely to require some such assistance. Late-life dependency of this kind does not create a corresponding demand on Medicare, however, because Medicare covers only a very small part of the costs of long-term care.

Another factor in the stereotypic image of the elderly as breaking the health care bank is the cost of medical treatment at the end of life. Medicare payments to people during their last year of life are substantial; they account for 27 to 30 percent of the annual Medicare budget. That proportion has not been increasing, however. Furthermore, end-of-life medical costs are lower for an older person than for a younger one.

This well-documented research finding, surprising at first glance, is readily explained. Eighty-year-old patients, compared to fifty-year-olds, are less likely to undergo major surgery, dialysis, and other invasive procedures. Their care is less resource-intensive and therefore less costly. For a sixty-nine-year-old who dies at age seventy, there is a $3,600 increase in health care costs during the last year of life, but for the eighty-nine-year-old who dies at age ninety, the increased cost of the final year is only $400. In short, once people reach age sixty-five, their additional years of life do not have a major effect on the costs of Medicare.

What *will* tend to drive up the costs of health care, at least until the year 2020 (when the baby boom generation hits sixty-five), is the relatively large number of baby boomers. The greatest potential savings in these future costs can come from prevention—that is, from improving the health-promotive lifestyle of middle-aged people today. Proper habits of diet, exercise, and nonsmoking, as we have seen, improve health and well-being whenever they are begun, but the earlier they are initiated, the greater are the lifetime savings in health costs. Old age is not the enemy of cost containment.

What They Give: Contributions of the Elderly

The image of the elderly as uniformly affluent—extravagant consumers of goods and services—is mistaken, as we have just seen. And the other aspect of the anti-elderly stereotype, the idea that older people do not produce and thus contribute little or nothing to the larger society, is also wrong.

As discussed in chapter 11, the underestimation of productivity in old age comes mainly from the economically convenient but conceptually inappropriate definition of productive activity as anything that is paid for, but nothing that is done without pay. Thus, the young man who makes a substantial living dealing blackjack in a casino is counted as productive, but the older woman who spends an equal number of hours as a volunteer in a hospital is counted as unproductive. As this example suggests, limiting the definition of productivity to work done for pay not only underestimates the total amount of productive work, it does so in an unequal fashion. More of the productive work done by older men and women is unpaid, and so the paid-work-only definition discriminates against them.

We gave productive activity a broader and more appropriate definition—any activity, paid or unpaid, that generates goods or services of economic value. When that definition is used, the statistics about the productivity of older people change dramatically.

If we include as productive work things of economic value that older people do for themselves, their families, and their friends, the percentage who are counted as productive goes still higher. More than 90 percent do some housework, more than 80 percent do home maintenance of other kinds, and 70 percent provide help of various kinds to friends and relatives.

ACTUAL AND POTENTIAL: PROSPECTS FOR INCREASED PRODUCTIVITY

Impressive as the actual contributions of older men and women are, their potential contributions are still greater. Moreover, many of the signs are favorable for realizing that potential. First, there is capacity; although almost one in three older people do some volunteer work, at least two out of three do none. Moreover, most of those who volunteer do so for very few hours. Estimates vary, but most older volunteers work between one and four hours per week.

Second, the values and attitudes of older people are favorable to volunteerism. At least eight out of ten say they agree with such statements as "Older people who no longer can work should contribute through community service" or "Life is not worth living if one cannot contribute to the well-being of others."

Third, substantial numbers of people who do not volunteer say they are "willing and able."

Fourth, older people have an apparent ability for and interest in paid work, as well as in volunteering. Nine percent of all men and women fifty-five to sixty-four years of age are not working for pay, but are willing and able to do so. That percentage increases to thirteen among people aged sixty-five to seventy-four, and even among those age seventy-five and older, 8 percent report themselves as willing and able to work (for pay). To put it in terms of potential additions to current employment, the gains would be about 20 percent in the fifty-five- to sixty-four-year group, 80 percent in the sixty-five- to seventy-four-year group, and 200 percent (!) in the oldest (seventy-five-plus) group.

In short, by any available measure, older men and women are an underutilized productive resource. The great challenge to policy makers and leaders of organizations is how best to tap the experience, energy, and motivation of older people.

REALIZING THE POTENTIAL: WHAT WILL IT TAKE?

When Einstein was asked to comment on the significance of the atom bomb, he said sadly, "It has changed everything . . . everything but our way of thinking," and went on to explain the danger of that great gap between the new reality and the old ideas of national supremacy and war as a means of attaining it. Changes in the age structure of society, in life expectancy and sustained ability, have been less dramatic, but scarcely less profound in their effects. And as with the advent of the nuclear age, our ways of thinking about aging have yet to catch up with the new realities. The stakes in that great game of societal catch-up are very high.

In this section we discuss three specific areas in which change must occur—concepts of the life course, methods of social accounting, and the allocation of education, work, and leisure.

CONCEPTS OF THE LIFE COURSE

The United States is what sociologists call an "age-graded society." Largely on the basis of age, our customs, our laws, and our institutions tell people what they can and can't do. There is an age at which children must go to school and an age before which they cannot leave; there is an age at which young people may legally drink alcoholic beverages, an age at which they can vote, and an age at which they can join the armed forces. Until recently, there was an age at which retirement became mandatory, and there is an age at which people become eligible for Social Security benefits. That, however, is the end of age grading; the years of retirement are blank. As Ernest Burgess put it long ago, old age is a roleless role, a time of life when nothing is expected of you. That lack of structure is both a gift and a burden; we are reminded of the small child in the ultraprogressive nursery school who asked plaintively, "Do we have to do what we want to do again today?"

Admittedly, many older people find the absence of formal obligations welcome in some ways. At the societal level, however, it reflects a way of thinking that is obsolete, the idea that over sixty-five is over the hill. When Bismarck startled late nineteenth-century Germany with the proposal that workers over sixty-five years of age should receive a pension from the government, sixty-five was indeed over the hill. Most people did not live to that age, and most of those who did had little time left. Our situation, as we have seen, is much different—but our way of thinking about life after sixty-five has yet to recognize those differences.

Almost twenty years ago, gerontologist Bernice Neugarten,

recognizing that the undifferentiated designation of everyone over sixty-five as old was inappropriate, proposed a distinction between the young-old and old-old. Neugarten's two-stage model of aging described the young-old as relatively healthy, having an adequate income, and maintaining close relationships with relatives and friends. The old-old were more likely to be confronting serious symptoms of disease and disability, to be feeling financial strain, and to be relatively lonely and isolated. The young-old/old-old dichotomy has become part of the gerontological vocabulary, sometimes elevated to a trichotomous distinction between young-old, middle-old, and old-old, corresponding to ages fifty-five to sixty-five, sixty-five to seventy-five, and over seventy-five.

Others have gone still farther and have proposed a view of the life course as consisting of four quarters, each about twenty-five years long. The first quarter is seen as devoted mainly to maturation and education, and the second quarter as a time of young adulthood in which the core activities are career development, household formation, and parenting. In the third quarter, beginning around age fifty, children are grown and leave the parental home, earnings are at or near maximum, and health is good. Finally, in the fourth quarter, activity reduces and health concerns increase.

Of course, not all men and women live into the fourth quarter, let alone to its completion at age 100, but the idea has much to recommend it. The quarter-century idea approximates the time of some major life transitions, and the identification of ages fifty to seventy-five as the third quarter of life, while admittedly on the optimistic side, comes closer to the emerging demographic realities. Introducing the span of fifty to seventy-five years also counters the long emphasis on age sixty-five, and reminds us that the retention of functions and vigorous life beyond that age is increasingly the norm rather than the exception. Furthermore, it is in the third-quarter age range that we are experiencing some of the most rapid population growth. In 1985, there were about 50 million people in this age group and they constituted about one-fifth of the population of the

United States; by 2010, that age group is estimated to be 85 million, nearly one-third of the total population. If we are to change our thinking about aging, the third quarter is a good place to begin.

METHODS OF SOCIAL ACCOUNTING

All productive activities count but not all are counted. The Decennial Census, the monthly reports of the Current Population Survey, and the news releases from the U.S. Department of Labor keep before the public the statistics on paid employment and unemployment. They tell us nothing, however, about the large numbers of unpaid volunteers on whom churches, hospitals, and civic organizations of all kinds depend. Nor do the official statistics tell us anything about the numbers of people who provide valuable services in less formal settings, by caring for friends or family members who are temporarily or permanently unable to care for themselves.

Much of what keeps our society glued together, in spite of its many divisive tendencies, is unpaid activity of these kinds. People who do these many important things are not motivated by pay, since they are not paid, but by their commitment to organizations, to "good causes," and most of all to other people. If these are their motives, why is it important to count their activities and estimate their value in monetary terms?

There are several answers to this question, all of them closely related. First, we have become, as computer gurus and futurologists remind us, an information society, a society in which accurate information is increasingly important. We spend billions of dollars to generate quantitative information about the state of our world; we count what we consider important and, circular as it may seem, we tend to consider important the things that we have counted. By not counting the forms and quantity of unpaid productive work, we designate it as relatively unimportant.

A second reason for counting unpaid work is that good data make for wise decisions. Data are no substitute for wisdom or for humane values, but they give these qualities a base from which to act.

Finally, as we saw in chapter 11, most of the productive work of older men and women is unpaid, whereas most work of younger people, especially younger men, is in the form of paid employment. It follows that failure to count unpaid productive activity is not merely an underestimation of the effort by which our society functions; it is an underestimation that is biased against older people. Their major mode of contribution becomes officially invisible. To the extent that public perceptions and policy decisions are data based or data influenced, they are biased against the elderly.

For all these reasons, government statistics should treat unpaid work like paid employment; that is, its hours, type, location, and market value should be reported at regular intervals. The value of that work should then be included as a separately identified component of the Gross Domestic Product (GDP). Those who perform such work would thus be identified as societal contributors rather than burdens. That in turn may lead to an increase in the opportunities and invitations to voluntary activity and an increase in the motivation of older people to engage in it. In short, bringing our official information gathering and reporting into line with the changing facts of demography, the increasing numbers of older people, and their present and potential contributions will be both a sign that our thinking is changing and a means of continuing the change.

THE CHALLENGE OF INSTITUTIONAL CHANGE

To alter the allocation of education, work, and leisure over the life course is to take on the challenge of institutional change. Such changes tend to be incremental, and that is probably fortunate. It is important, however, for those gradual changes to be informed by a vision or goal that gives them direction and provides a basis for assessing their accomplishments. Our vision for a society in which people are encouraged and enabled to age successfully cannot be achieved for the elderly alone; it involves the entire life course and the major life activities that define it. We need to think about the life course in new ways, and then identify both the barriers that prevent American society from moving toward that new ideal and the incentives toward its realization. In the remainder of this chapter, we discuss these issues and conclude with a proposal for the reorganization of work throughout the life course.

Education, Work, and Leisure

Matilda and John Riley, veteran gerontologists who have been long concerned with such issues, have dramatized them by describing two extreme types of society, one in which major life roles are completely determined by age and the other in which age is entirely irrelevant. In the first of these hypothetical societies, the one that is wholly age-segregated, education would be only for children and adolescents, work (paid employment) would be only for young and (early) middle-aged adults, and leisure would be entirely for men and women beyond the retirement age. In the second imaginary society, which the Rileys call age-integrated, age is wholly irrelevant to major life activity; the allocation of education, work, and leisure is the same for people of all ages.

No thoughtful person would advocate either extreme, and certainly the authors do not. The complete restriction of education to the early years of life and the limitation of leisure to the late years are equally unappealing. The spectacle of child labor at one end of the life course and work without the possibility of retirement at the other end is even more offensive to contemplate. Nevertheless, the two hypothetical extremes serve their several purposes: they make it clear that our aspirations for society lie somewhere between the extremes and they remind us that American society at present is more age-segregated than age-integrated. They remind us also that the earlier history of the United States, like that of other countries when they were struggling with the transition from agricultural to industrial dominance, was a time in which education was limited, work continued to the point of physical frailty, and life beyond that point was brief.

Let us think of the allocation of education, work, and leisure at three historical periods—past, present, and future. In the past, say, at the end of the nineteenth century or earlier, life was relatively short; formal education for most people was restricted to a few childhood years; work was almost lifelong, and leisure was minimal except in extreme old age and disability.

At present, here at the end of the twentieth century, people have a much longer life span, a considerably longer period of formal education during youth, and a greatly increased period of leisure in late-middle and old age (presumably after formal retirement). Children and adolescents have somewhat more leisure, although it is more organized than at earlier periods. And men and women have a great deal more leisure during the long years of retirement. Leisure during the formal working years is still very limited, especially when children are young. And opportunity for adult education, some of it job-related and some more broadly liberal, has increased.

Finally, we can imagine a future in which there is a substantial increase in lifelong education, a comparable increase in leisure time during the years of employment and child-rearing, and a reduction in the years of complete retirement. Late life in this imagined future shows a mixed pattern—education continuing but diminishing, formal work also reducing but not vanishing, and leisure increasing gradually in old age.

If our hopeful vision for the future is, as we believe it to be, closer to what people need and better for society as a whole, an obvious question arises: why does America not move quickly toward bringing reality into line with that vision? The answer is not a general resistance to change. All of us witness continual changes in clothing, hair styling, and physical ornamentation. As this is written, we behold boys and young men suddenly wearing baseball caps and, as if on signal, rotating them so that the visor is at the back of the head instead of the front. Young women, meanwhile, have progressed from single to multiple earrings and have moved on to the dutiful piercing of more sensitive and less visible body parts. By the time this is read, other fashions will have become equally popular. The rapid succession of such fads suggests a persisting human appetite for change rather than an inborn resistance to it. And, at least in some sectors of society, there are the more encouraging signs of dietary changes and increases in other health-promotive activities.

BARRIERS TO CHANGE

The factors that oppose changes in the pattern of education, work, and leisure throughout the life course are of several types—psychological, organizational, and legal. The psychological opposition to allowing such changes comes from the stereotypes that many people still hold, the myths about what older men and women can and should do. (See chapter 1, Breaking Down the Myths of Aging.)

Organizational Barriers

These factors are even more important obstacles to changing the pattern of adult education, work, and leisure. Work schedules tend to be rigid; a full-time job is defined as eight hours a day and forty hours a week. Flexible arrangements are becoming more common, but most people feel that their choice as employees is all or nothing; the employing organization defines the job and the prospective employee must take it or leave it. It remains to be seen whether the recent organizational tendency to convert some jobs from conventional employment to "independent contracting" enables employees to define their own work schedules or merely deprives them of job security and fringe benefits.

Recent years have seen two other tendencies in the corporate world that have reduced opportunities for the employment of older workers—downsizing and early retirement inducements. Downsizing, as the coined term suggests, is a systematic reduction in the number of employees in an organization. The reduction may be triggered by any of several factors: technological developments that replace workers with computer-assisted machinery, corporate mergers that enable consolidation of previously competing organizational units, or changes in the organizational environment that compel new economies. Almost regardless of the reason for downsizing, it affects older workers disproportionately. This is partly because of the stereotypes that many managers hold but mainly because the seniority of older workers is an organizational cost; wages and salaries tend to be seniority-driven.

Recent national legislation has made compulsory retirement for reasons of age alone illegal, although many older workers nevertheless feel pressure to retire. Others, more fortunate, are offered financial inducements to do so. Especially in the professional and managerial ranks, these arrangements have become common enough to have generated a new terminology—golden parachutes, golden handshakes, and the like.

The traditional formalities of higher education must also be counted among the organizational barriers to a more age-integrated society. Colleges and universities have been slow to adjust their schedules and requirements to encourage intermittent or sustained course work by adults of all ages. Most colleges and universities act as if they prefer full-time students in residence, working uninterruptedly toward one or another academic degree and completing the requirements within the prescribed number of years—four years for a bachelor's degree, one or two additional for a master's degree. There are signs of increasing flexibility on the institutional fringes of universities, however—programs of learning in retirement, courses scheduled on weekends and in evenings, for example. Perhaps more important, community colleges, a rapidly growing sector of educational institutions, have concentrated on serving people whose age, academic credentials, or responsibilities make standard university curricula and degree programs inappropriate.

Legal Barriers

All the preceding barriers to achieving greater integration of education, work, and leisure activities across the life course are erected, strengthened, weakened, or removed within a context of laws, executive rulings, and court decisions. For the most part, these legal factors, operating mainly at state and national levels, have limited rather than facilitated the attainment of optimal patterns of the three major life activities. Recent years, however, have seen the lowering of some of the most important legal barriers.

First among such barrier reductions was the abolition of mandatory retirement for reasons of age; the law ended age-mandated retirement for most occupations in 1986 and it was extended to almost all occupations in 1994. Second in importance was the change in the federal income tax law that lowered the age at which people receiving Social Security pensions could also earn additional income without forfeiting pension income, and increased the level at which earned income effectively reduced pension income.

A third economic factor, part legislative and part quasilegal, is the tendency of pension formulas themselves to favor retirement rather than continued employment. Economists argue that both Social Security and company pension arrangements have not been actuarially neutral. For example, one year of paid employment before the formal retirement age generates both direct wage or salary income and increased pension entitlements (through employer contributions and tax-deferred employee contributions). In many pension systems, however, a year of employment after the age at which retirement is allowed does not add proportionately to the amount of the pension. Moreover, the person who continues to work for additional years loses the pension income for those years. The actuarial computations are complex and most people certainly have not performed them. Nevertheless, people act as if they understood such trade-offs; they tend to retire when it is in their economic interests to do so.

FACTORS FAVORING CHANGE

More important than the barriers to change, we now look at the factors which *promote* change.

Psychological Factors

The persisting time pressures of employment, homemaking, and parenting in the two-job family have generated a wish for fewer hours of paid work, even with a commensurate reduction in income. Offered this hypothetical trade-off, 51 percent of women and 42 percent of men preferred more time with family and less at work.

The underlying attitudes of older people themselves toward continuing productive activity are mixed; the majority believe that older people should contribute to society as long as they are able, but they also believe that older people have "earned the right to leisure." The implication is for some combination of continued work (but less than full-time) and increased leisure.

Informational Factors

There seems to be increasing public awareness that most older people are healthy and able to contribute productively, and there is certainly increased public sensitivity, partly misguided, about the entitlements of older people. The chronic overwork of younger adults, the need for recurrent job-related education as people age and technology changes, and the importance of diplomas and college degrees for young people entering the labor market are also becoming more widely recognized.

Organizational Factors

Some organizations, but still a minority, permit phased retirement, some permit substantial hours of work at home, and some substitute consulting agreements and "independent contracting" for conventional full-time employment. To the extent that such arrangements are successful and become widely known, they encourage flexibility more broadly.

Legal and Governmental Factors

In recent years, public policies affecting employment of older people have shifted from antiwork to neutral. Most important were the successive increases in the age of mandatory retirement and its virtual elimination in 1994. Beginning in 1983, earnings limits for people receiving Social Security payments were raised for all recipients and were eliminated for those age seventy and above. In addition, the financial incentives for delaying retirement are being gradually increased; by the year 2010, each year of delayed retirement will increase a person's Social Security stipend by 8 percent.

Other federal legislation sets goals, but their fulfillment depends on annual budgetary decisions by Congress. For example, several sections of the Older Americans Act, which dates from 1965, include such aims as encouraging productive roles among older people (Title IV) and facilitating the employment of low-income older people in community service (Title V).

POLICIES FOR THE FUTURE: GETTING FROM HERE TO THERE

Suppose that we in the United States were to agree that we wanted a better combination of activities throughout the life course, that the compartmentalized pattern of activities at different ages is no longer in the national interest. We would be agreed on our goal and would then have to discover or invent the means to attain it. We would, in short, confront the classic question of any planned change: how do we get from here to there?

Here are three promising possibilities.

LEARNING FROM THE JAPANESE EXAMPLE

In the 1980s, responding belatedly to the remarkable Japanese success in improving the quality of automobiles and electronic equipment, American manufacturers decided to learn from their major international competitor. Neither the competition nor the learning process is at an end, but it has become mutual and, on the whole, beneficial.

Since life expectancy in Japan is even greater than in the United States, and since the Japanese birth rate is significantly lower than ours, Japanese policy makers have confronted earlier than we the problem of how to encourage paid and voluntary activity among older people. Three resulting developments contribute to the solution—the concept of postretirement careers, direct governmental subsidies to private employers, and the creation of Silver Manpower Centers.

The Japanese concept of working at well-defined successive jobs in a gradual march toward complete retirement is perhaps most obvious in the educational sector. Professors in major universities "retire" from one institution and are appointed at another, typically one in which their specialty is less fully developed and in which their own role may be less demanding. The pattern is followed in other occupations as well. The Japanese government provides subsidies to private companies that encourage this process. Such subsidies are given to companies that hire older workers, age fifty-five to sixty-four, who have been retired from other organizations. Companies that reassign their own "retired" workers, age sixty to sixty-four, to full-time or part-time jobs are also subsidized for doing so.

The Silver Manpower Centers are agencies that attempt to match older people to productive activities, either paid or voluntary. The centers themselves began as voluntary organizations in 1975, but in 1985 a law was passed that made their establishment official and allocated government funds for their support. Their goals were lofty: help promote a wholesome, meaningful life for older people, encourage their participation in community life, and assist them in the transition from work to retirement. The law also set the community goal of utilizing the experience of the elderly. Some economic support was provided to the Silver Manpower Centers, but the means for realizing their goals emphasized "self-organization" and the sharing of work. The centers reported that 60 percent of the older people enrolled in their programs found work.

WHAT GOVERNMENT CAN DO

The Silver Manpower Centers of Japan illustrate some things government can do by direct allocation of resources, but governments can also affect the mix of education, work, and leisure by altering the regulations under which private organizations function and by providing new information to the public. The following are examples of what the United States government can do, based on these three categories.

Direct Allocation of Resources

Almost every session of Congress debates one or more proposals on the direct allocation of resources to older people. Direct educational subsidies, like those offered to returning veterans after World War II, can certainly stimulate increased enrollment in post-secondary school training. The government could also separate health insurance from employment, thus enabling people to make choices about retirement, part-time employment, or educational leave without loss of health coverage. A change of this kind, however, implies a shifting of health insurance costs from employers to government.

Government could also allocate funds to encourage voluntary activity. Funds could be used to create and publicize voluntary programs in areas not already served, and also to provide stipends to volunteers. The concept of a stipend-volunteer program is not a contradiction in terms; the main purpose of such stipends is to offset the expenses of volunteering—transportation, accident and liability insurance, and the like. Low-income volunteers might also receive a modest stipend as token earnings. At least four federally supported stipend-volunteer programs are already in operation: the Retired Senior Volunteer Program (RSVP), the Senior Companion Program, the Foster Grandparent Program, and the Service Corps of Retired Executives (SCORE).

Changes in Employer Regulations

Many possible regulatory changes could create more flexibility in the lifelong mix of education, employment, and leisure *without* direct resource allocation by government. For example, making entitlement to fringe benefits such as employer pension contributions, life insurance, and educational leave proportional to the number of hours worked would make it easier for employers to hire part-time workers and for workers to move from full-time to part-time work without disproportionate losses in benefits. Many benefit programs now operate with a kind of all-or-nothing rule, which means that employees who work more than some stipulated fraction—half-time or three-quarters time, for example—are entitled to full benefits, while those who work fewer hours have no benefit entitlement.

Improving the Information Base

The federal government is the primary source of information about employment and unemployment, about the performance of the national economy, and many other factors that describe the overall quality of American life. As we saw in chapter 11, these statistics tell us a great deal about paid employment, but almost nothing about unpaid productive work. The result is a persistent underestimation of the activities that maintain American society. Moreover, since unpaid work is more prominent in the lives of women than men, and more prominent in the lives of older people than younger, statistics that fail to count unpaid productive work are biased against women and the elderly. Continuing to gather data on the work of volunteers, on hours spent in providing care to family members and friends, and the like, can counter the stereotypic image of aging, and correct the mistaken impression that the elderly are a burden to the rest of society.

THE WORK MODULE

We propose that paid employment be organized on the basis of four-hour modules. The purpose of the four-hour module is to increase flexibility in work arrangements, to enable older people to choose a gradual transition from full-time employment to retirement, and younger people to choose family or educational time over work time when it suits their needs to do so. The work module is *not* a proposal to reduce hours of work overall or to redefine four hours as a full day's work. On the contrary, the probable effect of introducing this work module would be to increase total hours of paid work, largely through increased labor force participation of older men and women.

A work module is simply a time-task unit, the smallest allocation of time that is economically and psychologically meaningful for performing a given task. To meet these criteria, we assume that a module of four hours would be generally appropriate—four hours operating a drill press, working at a computer, waiting tables in a restaurant, or seeing patients in a hospital emergency room. (Health care has already begun this approach—many physicians have their workweek divided into half-day or four-hour "sessions," with the usual week including eight patient care sessions and the remainder dedicated increasingly to teaching, reading to keep up to date, and paperwork.)

It is obvious that a conventional eight-hour-a-day, five-day-a-week job, full-time by the current definition, would consist of two such modules per day, ten per week and, assuming a brief two-week vacation, 500 per year. But there is nothing sacred about that pattern. At the beginning of this century, a full-time job meant six days and sixty hours each week. Furthermore, the forty-hour week no longer coincides, if it ever did, with the work schedules of organizations. Most organizations do not operate on the basis of eight-hour days and five-day weeks. Factories may run two or three shifts; hospitals must provide many services on a twenty-four-hour basis, and many supermarkets do the same; department stores and retail malls are open most evenings, seven days a week. The use of the four-hour work module would not significantly add to such costs.

Increased individual choice about hours of work would take many forms and satisfy all age groups. For the large numbers of older employees who prefer it, phased retirement would replace the present unsatisfactory choice between all or nothing. For the still larger number of younger men and women who say that they would prefer the financial sacrifice of fewer hours of work in exchange for more time with family, the work module offers them that possibility. As early as 1977, in households with both parents present and children aged seventeen or less, almost half of the parents said they would chose family time over money.

As these examples imply, the four-hour work module does not imply a workday of only four hours, or a workweek of twenty. Some people would prefer longer workdays, and fewer of them each week. Some would want a period of intensive work, followed by a semester's leave for full-time education. The use of the four-hour work module is to accommodate such changing needs, not to substitute a new rigidity for an old one.

The concept of the work module rests on a simple proposition: that individuals already know, or can discover, the combination of employment, education, and other activity that best suits their needs. These needs are different for different individuals and they change for everyone as people age, external demands ebb and flow, and new opportunities present themselves. A person's initial choice, therefore, would not be permanently binding; it would likely change, although not so frequently as to disrupt the performance of a work group or the organization as a whole.

Were people to be given the opportunity to define the time pattern of their employment in this way, the immediate effect should be increased satisfaction with the job itself. Effects on health should also be positive, since improvement in goodness-of-fit between the person and the job means reduction in job stress. And the effects on other major life roles—as spouse, parent, student, friend, citizen—would also likely be positive. Effects on the larger community would be harder to trace, but we would expect them to be significant. Paid employment, as we have seen, is only one of the forms of productive activity on which communities and societies depend. Others include unpaid work and participation in voluntary organizations, informal assistance to others, and care of one's home and family. To the extent that increased flexibility in paid employment frees time for other productive activities, the quality of community life is enhanced.

The work organizations, corporate and governmental, that adopted the work module would incur the costs of creating and maintaining a somewhat more complex procedure for work scheduling. But those costs would be more than offset, we believe, by reductions in absence and turnover, and by the increased loyalty and work motivation of employees.

That we need better allocation of paid employment, education, and other activities throughout the life course is clear. The policies and procedures best suited to achieve those goals are not equally clear. The work module is one proposal for their attainment, one approach to improving the integration of work, education, and leisure to which we aspire. In short, it is a hypothesis rather than a conclusion. It is a hypothesis based on a great deal of research but, like all hypotheses, it requires testing before it is adopted as policy.

The evaluation of serious policy proposals requires experimental trials on a scale large enough to be persuasive and small enough so that mistakes are not too costly. Such an experimental approach is novel only in its application to problems of social policy. In corporate life, it is familiar as the pilot plant and in medicine, as the clinical trial.

The United States itself, established more than 200 years ago with an unprecedented democratic structure, has been called a social experiment. Donald Campbell proposed that to solve the complex policy problems of our own time, we would also have to become "an experimenting society," a society that tests major new policies on a limited basis and modifies them as necessary before adopting them more generally. Nothing less will suffice to move us successfully toward a better integration of life's major activities—paid employment, education and reeducation, homemaking and parenting, voluntarism and informal support, and leisure. The better integration of these activities over the life course will, in turn, make successful aging more attainable for all of us.

NOTES

INTRODUCTION
Sources of Statistical Information

Bell, F., et al. Life Tables for the United States 1900–2080. Actuarial Study No. 107. Washington, DC: Social Security Administration Publication 11-11536.

Byerly, E.R. (1993). State Population Estimates by Age and Sex: 1980 to 1992. Washington, DC: U.S. Bureau of the Census, Current Population Reports, Series P25, No. 1106.

Day, J.C. (1992). Population projections of the United States, by Age, Sex, Race, and Hispanic Origin. Current Population Reports, Series P-25, No. 1092.

Dublin, L.I., et al. (1949). *Length of life: study of the life table.* New York: Ronald Press Co.

Fowles, D.G. (1991). *A profile of older Americans: 1990.* Washington, DC: American Association of Retired Persons and Administration of Aging, U.S. Dept of Health and Human Services.

Lee, R.D., et al. (1992). Modeling and forecasting United States mortality. *Journal of the American Statistical Association* 87(419):659.

Linder, F.E., et al. (1947). Vital Statistics Rates in the United States, 1900–1940. Washington, DC: Government Printing Office.

Sutherland, J.E., et al. (1990): Proportionate mortality trends: 1950 through 1986. *Journal of the American Medical Association* 264:3178.

Torrey, B.B., et al. An aging world. Washington, DC: U.S. Bureau of the Census, *International Population Reports,* Series P-95, No. 78.

U.S. Bureau of the Census (1996). Current Population Reports, Special Studies, P23-190, 65+ in the United States. Washington, DC: Government Printing Office.

Recommended Scholarly Articles

Austad, S.N. (1977). *Why we age.* New York: Wiley.

Brody, J.A. (1995). Postponement as prevention in aging. In Butler, R., and Brody, J.A., eds., *Strategies to delay dysfunction in later life.* New York: Springer.

Brody, J.A., et al. (1987). Trends in the health of the elderly population. *Annual Review of Public Health* 8:211.

Carnes, B.A., et al. (1993). Evolutionary perspectives on human senescence. *Population Development Review* 19:793.

Crimmins, E.M., et al. (1997). Further evidence on recent trends in the prevalence and incidence of disability among older Americans from two sources: the LSOA and the NHIS. *Journal of Gerontology: Social Sciences* 52B(2), 559.

Furner, S.E., et al. (1994). The aging population. In O'Donnell, P.D., ed., *Geriatric urology.* Boston: Little, Brown & Company.

Manton, K.G., et al. (1996). Longevity in the United States: age and sex-specific evidence on life span limits from mortality patterns 1960–1990. *Journal of Gerontology: Biological Sciences* 51A:B362.

———. (1997). Chronic disability trends in elderly United States populations, 1982–1994. *Proceedings of the National Academy of Science* 94:2593.

Martin, L.G., et al. (1997). *Racial and ethnic differences in the health of older Americans.* Washington, DC: National Academy Press.

Olshansky, S.J., et al. (1986). The fourth stage of the epidemiologic transition: the age of delayed degenerative diseases. *Milbank Quarterly* 64:355.

———. (1990). In search of Methuselah: estimating the upper limits to human longevity. *Science* 250:634.

Preston, S. (1992). *The oldest old.* New York: Oxford University Press.

Rogers, R., et al. (1989). Extending epidemiologic transition theory: a new stage. *Social Biology* 34(3–4):234.

Verbrugge, L.M. (1989). The dynamics of population aging and health. In Lewis, S.J., ed., *Aging and health: linking research and public policy.* Chelsea, MI: Lewis Publishers.

Wetle, T. (1997). Living longer, aging better. *Journal of the American Medical Association* 278:1376.

NOTE: It is important to clarify our use of the terms "senescence" and "aging." In scientific terms, one's age is a measure of the number of years one has lived. Since aging occurs as a function of the additional years since birth, strictly speaking everyone ages at the same rate. Senescence, on the other hand, refers to the biological and physiological changes that occur in an individual as he or she ages. Senescence is highly variable, and proceeds at different rates in different people. The term "aging" is often used, in this book and elsewhere, interchangeably with senescence to describe the changes in the function and health status of individuals or society as their age increases. As will be discussed in detail later in this book, the MacArthur Foundation's Research Studies on Successful Aging have conclusively shown that differences in the rate of senescence are related not only to genetic factors, but also to a number of lifestyle factors that importantly influence the rate at which our bodies change with advancing age. In sum, how successfully one ages is largely determined by how hard one works at it throughout life.

CHAPTER I
Myth 1: "To Be Old Is to Be Sick"

Butler, R.N. (1975). *Why survive? Being old in America*. New York: Harper & Row.

Crimmins, E., et al. (1989). Changes in life expectancy and disability-free life expectancy in the United States. *Population Development Review* 15:235.

Dychtwald, K. (1989). *Age wave—the challenges and opportunities of an aging America*. Los Angeles: J.P. Tarcher.

Freedman, V.A., et al., eds. (1994). Trends in disabilities at older ages. Committee of National Statistics, National Research Council. Washington, DC: National Academy Press.

Friedan, B. (1993). *The fountain of age*. New York: Simon and Schuster.

Fries, J.F. (1980). Aging, natural death and the compression of morbidity. *New England Journal of Medicine* 303:130.

———. (1989). The compression of morbidity: near or far? *Milbank Quarterly* 67:208.

Guralnik, J.M., et al. (1995). The Women's Health and Aging Study: health and social characteristics of older women with disability. Bethesda, MD: National Institute on Aging, National Institutes of Health publication no. 95-4009.

Holmes, O.W. (1861). "The deacon's masterpiece or the wonderful one-horse shay." In *Poems. 20th edition*. Boston: Ticknor & Fields.

———. (1893). *"The one-horse shay," with its companion poems*. Boston: Houghton Mifflin.

Manton, K.G., et al. (1993). Estimates of change in chronic disability and institutionalization, incidence and prevalence rates in the United States elderly population from the 1992, 1984, and 1989 National Long-Term Care Surveys. *Journal of Gerontology* 48:S153.

————. (1995). Changes in morbidity and chronic disability in the U.S. elderly population; evidence from the 1982, 1984, and 1989 National Long-Term Care Surveys. *Journal of Gerontology* 50:S194.

————. (1997). Chronic disability trends in elderly United States population, 1982–1994. *Proceedings of National Academy of Science* 94:2593.

Olshansky, S.J., et al. (1991). Trading off longer life for worsening health: the expansion of morbidity hypothesis. *Journal of Aging and Health* 3(2):194.

Preston, S. (1992). *The oldest old*. NY: Oxford University Press.

Robine, J.M., et al. (1991). Healthy life expectancy: evaluation of a new global indicator of change in population health. *British Medical Journal* 302:457.

Rogers, R., et al. (1989). Active life expectancy among the elderly in the United States: multi-state life-table estimates and population projection. *Milbank Quarterly* 67:370.

Rowe, J.W. (1997). The new gerontology. *Science* 278:367.

Rudberg, M., et al. (1993). Are death and disability in old age preventable? In Albarede, J.L., Garry, P.J., and Vallas, D., eds., *Facts and research in gerontology*, Springer (USA) 7:191.

Trends in the Health of Older Americans; United States 1994 (April 1995). National Center for Health Statistics, U.S. Department of Health and Human Services, Center for Disease Control and Prevention.

Verbrugge, L.M. (1984). Longer life but worsening health? Trends in health and mortality of middle-aged and older persons. *Milbank Quarterly* 62:475.

Myth 2: "You Can't Teach an Old Dog New Tricks"

American Health (May 1997):95.

Burack, O.R., et al. (1996). The effects of list-making on recall in young and elderly adults. *Journals of Gerontology, Series B: Psychological and Social Sciences* 51B(4), 226.

Kliegl, R., et al. (1989). Testing-the-limits and the study of adult age differences in cognitive plasticity of a mnemonic skill. *Developmental Psychology* 25, 247.

Schrank, H.T., et al. (1983). Aging and work organizations. In Riley, M.W., et al., eds., *Aging in society*, 53. Hillsdale, NJ: Erlbaum.

Myth 3: "The Horse Is Out of the Barn"

Cigarette Smoking

Hermanson, B., et al. (1988). Beneficial six-year outcome of smoking cessation in older men and women with coronary artery disease. *New England Journal of Medicine* 319:1365.

Higgins, M.W., et al. (1993). Smoking and lung function in elderly men and women. *Journal of the American Medical Association* 269:2741.

Syndrome X

Despres, J.P., et al. (1996). Hyperinsulinemia as an independent risk factor for ischemic heart disease. *New England Journal of Medicine* 334:952.

Foster, D.W., (1989). Insulin resistance—a secret killer (editorial). *New England Journal of Medicine* 320:733.

Katzel, L.I., et al. (1995). Effects of weight loss vs. aerobic exercise training on risk factors for coronary disease in healthy, obese, middle-aged, and older men. *Journal of the American Medical Association* 274:1915.

Zavaroni, I., et al. (1986). Effect of age and environmental factors on glucose tolerance and insulin secretion in a worker population. *Journal of the American Geriatrics Society* 34:271.

High Blood Pressure

(1991). Prevention of stroke by antihypertensive drug treatment in older persons with isolated systolic hypertension. Final results of the Systolic Hypertension in the Elderly Program (SHEP). *Journal of the American Medical Association* 265:3255.

Physical Fitness

Blair, S.N., et al. (1992). How much physical activity is good for health? *Annual Review of Public Health* 13:99.

———. (1995). Changes in physical fitness and all-cause mortality: a prospective study of healthy and unhealthy men. *Journal of the American Medical Association* 273:1093.

———. (1996). Influences of cardiorespiratory fitness and other precursors on cardiovascular disease and all-cause mortality in men and women. *Journal of the American Medical Association* 276:205.

Seeman, T., et al. (1994). Predicting changes in physical functioning in a high-functioning elderly cohort: MacArthur studies of successful aging. *Journal of Gerontology* 49:M97.

———. (1995). Behavioral and psychosocial predictors of physical performance: MacArthur studies of successful aging. *Journal of Gerontology* 50A:M177.

Sticht, J.P., et al. (1995). Weight control and exercise: cardinal features of successful preventative gerontology (editorial). *Journal of the American Medical Association* 274:1964.

Myth 4: "The Secret to Successful Aging Is to Choose Your Parents Wisely"

Cohen, B.H. (1964). Familial patterns of mortality and life span. *Quarterly Review of Biology* 39:130.

Finch, C.E. (1990). *Longevity, senescence and the genome.* Chicago: University of Chicago Press.

Finch, C.E., et al. (1997). Genetics of Aging. *Science* 278:407.

Hauge, M., et al. (1968). The Danish Twin Register. *Acta genetica medica gemellol* 17:315.

Heller, D.A., et al. (1993). Genetic and environmental influences on serum lipid levels in twins. *New England Journal of Medicine* 328:1150.

Hong, Y., et al. (1994). Genetic and environmental influences on blood pressure in elderly twins. *Hypertension* 24 (6):663.

Jarvik, L.F., et al. (1960). Survival trends in senescent twin populations. *American Journal of Human Genetics* 12:170.

Kallman, F.J., et al. (1959). Individual differences and constitution in genetic background. In Birren, J.E., ed., *Handbook of aging and the individual*, 216. Chicago: University of Chicago Press.

Martin, G.M. (1985). Genetics of human disease, longevity and aging. In Andres, R., Bierman, E.L., and Hazzard W.R., eds., *Principles of geriatric medicine*. New York: McGraw-Hill.

McClearn, G., et al. (1994). Genetic and environmental influences on pulmonary function in aging Swedish twins. *Journal of Gerontology* 49:M264.

——— (1997). Substantial genetic influence on cognitive abilities in twins 80 or more years old. *Science* 276:1560.

Pearl, R., et al. (1934). *The ancestry of the long lived.* London: Milford.

Stunkard, A.J., et al. (1990). The body-mass index of twins who have been reared apart. *New England Journal of Medicine* 322:1483.

Wachter, K.W. and Finch, Caleb E., eds. (1997). *Between Zeus and the salmon.* Washington: National Academy Press.

Two major forms of the "progeria" syndrome have been identified: Werner's syndrome, which develops after puberty and represents "adult onset" progeria, and a childhood form, the Hutchinson-Gilford syndrome, which begins in early childhood.

Myth 5: "The Lights May Be On, but the Voltage Is Low"

Cicero, M.T. (1744). *Cato major, or his discourse of old age: with explanatory notes.* Philadelphia: B. Franklin.

Kinsey, A.C. (1948). *Sexual behavior in the human male.* Philadelphia: W. B. Saunders Co.

———. (1953). *Sexual behavior in the human female.* Philadelphia: W. B. Saunders Co.

Schanck, R.L. (1932). A study of a community and its groups and institutions conceived of as behaviors of individuals. *Psychological Monographs* 43 (2).

For an extensive list of references on this subject, see:

Birren, J.E. *Sexuality and aging: a selected bibliography.* Los Angeles: Ethel Percy Andrus Gerontology Center. This bibliography, first published in 1975, has been successively revised and updated.

See also:

Glass, T.A., et al. (1995). Change in productive activity in late adulthood: MacArthur studies of successful aging. *Journal of Gerontology: Social Sciences* 50B(2), S65.

Kahn, R.L. (1984). Productive behavior through the life course: an essay on the quality of life. *Human Resource Management* 23(1), 5.

Morgan, J.N. (1986). Unpaid productive activity over the life course. In Institute of Medicine/National Research Council, eds., *America's aging: productive roles in an older society.* Washington, DC: National Academy Press.

Pfeiffer, E. (1974). Sexuality in the aging individual. *Journal of the American Geriatrics Society,* 22(11), 481.

Segraves, R.T,. and Segraves, K.B. (1995). Human sexuality and aging. *Journal of Sex Education and Therapy* 21(2), 88.

Wharton, G.F. (1981). *Sexuality and aging: an annotated bibliography.* Metuchen, NJ: Scarecrow Press.

The findings cited are from several major national surveys, including:

Americans Changing Lives, conducted by the Survey Research Center of the University of Michigan and supported by the National Institute on Aging. Health and Retirement Study, also conducted by the Survey Research Center and supported by the National Institute on Aging.

Aging in the eighties: America in transition. Washington, DC: National Council on Aging. (Survey data from Louis Harris and Associates.)

Myth 6: "The Elderly Don't Pull Their Own Weight"

Commonwealth Fund. (1990). *Americans over 55 at work program* (Research Reports 1 & 2). New York, NY.

Commonwealth Fund. (November 1993). *The untapped resource.* New York, NY.

Other references dealing with productive activity in old age are shown for Chapter 11.

CHAPTER 2

Paige, L. (1993). *Maybe I'll pitch forever.* Lincoln, NE: University of Nebraska Press.

In the Foreword to Paige's autobiography "as told to David Lipman," John B. Holway describes Paige as "not only . . . an amazing athlete, he was one of the great American humorists, in the tradition of Mark Twain, Will Rogers, and Yogi Berra." Perhaps the most frequently quoted of his many aphorisms is the immortal advice "Don't look back. Something might be gaining on you."

The riddle of his age can now be answered, at least within a year or two. LeRoy Paige was born in 1905, more or less. He pitched his first professional game in 1926 and his last one in 1965, about the time of his 60th birthday! The first half of his remarkable career was spent in the Negro Leagues. Not until 1948, with his 44th birthday coming on, did he become the first African-American pitcher in the major leagues.

James, W. (1920). Letter to H.G. Wells, September 11, 1906. *Letters of William James*, vol. 2.

Defining Successful Aging

Roget, P.M. (1994). *The original Roget's thesaurus of English words and phrases.* United Kingdom: Longman Group.

White, M. (1992). *Stephen Hawking: a life in science.* New York: Dutton.

Hundreds of books have been written about Franklin Delano Roosevelt and many more contain his formal speeches, his "fireside chats," and his official papers. For a sense of how he, and his family and staff, dealt with his severe disability on a daily basis during the years of his presidency, we refer readers to one of the most recent biographies:

Goodwin, D. (1994). *No ordinary time: Franklin and Eleanor Roosevelt: the home front in World War II.* New York: Simon and Schuster.

Avoiding Disease and Disability

Khachaturian, Z.S., and Radebaugh, T.S., eds. (1997). *Alzheimer's disease: causes, diagnosis, treatment, and care.* Boca Raton, FL: CRC Press.

National Institute on Aging. (August 1995). *Alzheimer's disease and related dementias: biomedical update.* Washington, DC: Department of Health and Human Services.

Snowdon, D.A. (1997). Aging and Alzheimer's disease: lessons from the Nun Study. *The Gerontologist* 37(2), 150.

See also:

AHEAD. (1995). *Overview of the AHEAD Study.* Ann Arbor, MI: Institute for Social Research.

Crystal, H., et al. (1988). Clinico-pathologic studies in dementia: nondemented subjects with pathologically confirmed Alzheimer's disease. *Neurology* 38(11), 1682.

Strahan, G.W. (January 22, 1997). National Center for Health Statistics: Data from the National Health Interview Survey, reported in *Overview of the AHEAD Study* (1995). Ann Arbor, MI: Institute for Social Research. Reported in the *Washington Post.*

For purposes of comparison, selected data from the National Health Interview Study, provided by the National Center for Health Statistics, are also included.

Maintaining Mental and Physical Function

Bureau of the Census. (May 1995). *Statistical brief: sixty-five plus in the United States.* Washington, DC: U.S. Department of Commerce, Economics and Statistics Administration.

Ericsson, K.A. (1990). Peak performance and age: an examination of peak performance in sports. In Baltes, P.B., and Baltes, M.M., eds., *Successful aging: perspectives from the behavioral sciences,* 164. Cambridge, UK: Cambridge University Press.

Manton, K.G., and Stallard, E. (1996). Changes in health, mortality, and disability and their impact on long-term care needs. *Journal of Aging and Social Policy,* 7 (3/4), 25.

Schaie, K.W. (1990). The optimization of cognitive functioning in old age: predictions based on cohort-sequential and longitudinal data. In Baltes, P.B., and Baltes, M.M., eds., *Successful aging: perspectives from the behavioral sciences,* 94. Cambridge, UK: Cambridge University Press.

Schaie, K.W., and Willis, S.L. (1986). Can decline in adult intellectual functioning be reversed? *Developmental Psychology* 22(2), 223.

Continuing Engagement with Life

Cumming, E. (1961). *Growing old: the process of disengagement.* New York: Basic Books.

Freud, S. (March 19, 1908). Letter to his daughter Mathilde. In Freud, E., ed. (1960). *Letters of Sigmund Freud.* New York: Basic Books. This letter is reprinted in Sherline, R. (1994). *Love anyhow,* 85. New York: Timken.

House, J.S., and Kahn, R.L. (1985). Measures and concepts of social support. In Cohen, S., and Syme, S. Leonard, eds., *Social support and health*, 83. New York: Academic Press.

Kahn, R.L., et al. (1989). Age difference in productive activities. *Journal of Gerontology: Social Sciences* 44(4), S129.

Rowe, J.W. (October 17, 1997). The New Gerontology. *Science* 278:367.

Singh, N.A., et al. (1997). A randomized controlled trial of progressive resistance training in depressed elders. *Journal of Gerontology: Medical Sciences* 52A(1), M27.

Successful Aging or the Imitation of Youth?

This is typically Shavian advice—a nonagenarian telling younger people not to aspire to immortality, at least on this planet. I (RLK) remember it as part of an interview filmed, in the days before television, by Fox Movietone News for presentation in movie theaters. However, the massive literature by and about Shaw includes several collections of his pithy comments on life, society, and his fellow humans. Two of them, one published the year before he died and one compiled after his death, are:

Shaw, G.B. (1949). *The quintessence of G.B.S.: the wit and wisdom of Bernard Shaw.* London: Hutchinson.

————. (1990). *Shaw: interviews and recollections.* Iowa City, IA: University of Iowa Press.

Ryff, C.D. (1989). Beyond Ponce de Leon and life satisfaction: new directions in quest of successful aging. *International Journal of Behavioral Development* 12(1), 35.

For a discussion of the concept of successful aging as used by various authors, see:

Baltes, P.B., and Baltes, M.M., eds. (1990). *Successful aging: perspectives from the behavioral sciences.* New York: Cambridge University Press. Especially Chapter 1.

CHAPTER 3

Abbott, R.D., et al. (1987). Diabetes and the risk of stroke: the Honolulu heart program. *Journal of the American Medical Association* 257:949.

Allen, S.C. (1992). Aging and the respiratory system. In Brocklehurst, J.C., Tallis, R.C., and Fillert, H.M., eds., *Textbook of geriatric medicine and gerontology,* 739. New York: Churchill Livingstone.

Donahue, R.P., et al. (1987). Post-challenge glucose concentration and coronary heart disease in men of Japanese ancestry: Honolulu heart program. *Diabetes* 36:189.

Feller, I., et al. (1976). Baseline results of therapy for burn patients. *Journal of the American Medical Association* 236:1943.

Foster, D.W. (1989). Insulin resistance—a secret killer (editorial). *New England Journal of Medicine* 320:733.

Hazzard, W.R., et al. (1990). Preventative gerontology: strategies for attenuation of the chronic disease of aging. *Principles of geriatric medicine and gerontology*, 167. New York: McGraw-Hill.

Katzel, L.I., et al. (1995). Effects of weight loss vs. aerobic exercise training on risk factors for coronary disease in healthy, obese, middle-aged, and older men. *Journal of the American Medical Association* 274:1915.

Miller, R.A. (1996). The aging immune system: primer and prospectus. *Science* 273:70.

(1991). Prevention of stroke by antihypertensive drug treatment in older persons with isolated systolic hypertension. Final results of the Systolic Hypertension in the Elderly Program (SHEP). *Journal of the American Medical Association* 265:3255.

Pyorala, K. (1979). Relationship of glucose tolerance and plasma insulin to the incidence of coronary heart disease: results of two population studies in Finland. *Diabetes Care* 2:131.

Rowe, J.W. (1990). Toward successful aging: limitation of the morbidity associated with "normal" aging. *Principles of geriatric medicine and gerontology*, 2d ed., 138. New York: McGraw-Hill.

Rowe, J.W., et al. (1987). Human aging: Usual and successful. *Science* 237:143.

———. (1997). Successful aging. *Gerontologist* 37:433.

An additional consideration regarding the comparison of risk in younger and older persons relates to the fact that in older persons underlying systems, i.e., vascular tree or central nervous system, are likely to have been exposed, over time, to cumulative deleterious effects of modest, often subtle, increases in potentially harmful physiologic factors, i.e., blood pressure, glucose, insulin, cortisol, etc. Thus, the vascular tree or brain of an older individual may reflect cumulative effects of numerous, perhaps daily, insults. The cumulative impact of these deleterious effects has been termed allostatic load (McEwen and Stellar, 1993). As a result of the impaired *resilience* induced by this allostatic load with advancing age the tolerance of an individual for out-of-range physiological stimuli may be constrained and the risk of an adverse effect such as myocardial ischemia or cerebral vascular insufficiency may be increased. The risk of adverse effects from physiological abnormalities may increase with advancing age as allostatic load accumulates and the "safe operating ranges" shrink.

McEwen suggests that increased excursions of plasma cortisol may represent one example of the potential adverse effects of such allostatic load. In some aging individuals evening cortisol levels are consistently higher than is normally seen. Since cortisol in high levels is recognized as toxic for neurons, it is possible that the daily exposure to modest "excess" cortisol might have a cumulative deleterious effect on the central nervous system, reducing neuronal resilience and the capacity to respond to stress.

McEwen, B.S., et al. (1993). Stress and the individual. *Archives of Internal Medicine* 153:2093.

CHAPTER 4

Cohen, B.H. (1964). Familial patterns of mortality and life span. *Quarterly Review of Biology* 39:130.

Finch, C.E. (1990). *Longevity, senescence and the genome.* Chicago: University of Chicago Press.

Hauge, M., et al. (1968). The Danish Twin Register. *Acta genetica medica gemellol* 17:315.

Heller, D.A., et al. (1993). Genetic and environmental influences on serum lipid levels in twins. *New England Journal of Medicine* 328:1150.

Hong, Y., et al. (1994). Genetic and environmental influences on blood pressure in elderly twins. *Hypertension* 24 (6):663.

Jarvik, L.F., et al. (1960). Survival trends in senescent twin populations. *American Journal of Human Genetics* 12:170.

Kallman, E.J., et al. (1959). Individual differences and constitution in genetic background. In Birren, J.E., ed., *Handbook of aging and the individual,* 216. Chicago: University of Chicago Press.

Martin, G.M., (1985). Genetics of human disease, longevity and aging. In Andres, R., Bierman, E.L., and Hazzard, W.R., eds., *Principles of geriatric medicine.* New York: McGraw-Hill.

McClearn, G., et al. (1994). Genetic and environmental influences on pulmonary function in aging Swedish twins. *Journal of Gerontology* 49:M264.

———. (1997). Substantial genetic influence on cognitive abilities in twins 80 or more years old. *Science* 276:1560.

Pearl, R., et al. (1934). *The ancestry of the long lived.* London: Milford.

Stunkard, A.J., et al. (1990). The body-mass index of twins who have been reared apart. *New England Journal of Medicine* 322:1483.

Zavaroni, I., et al. (1986). Effect of age and environmental factors on glucose tolerance and insulin secretion in a worker population. *Journal of the American Geriatrics Society* 34:271.

Interaction of nature and nurture—Perhaps the most widely recognized and best understood example of environmental influence on expression of a genetic abnormality is phenylketonuria, also termed PKU. The first inherited metabolic disorder to be identified, PKU was described by Folling in 1934. This disease occurs in approximately one in 20,000 individuals of Northern European descent and is due to an inherited abnormality in the metabolism of an amino acid—phenylalanine, widely found in normal diets.

All individuals have a paired set of genes for the enzyme that normally breaks down phenylalanine. Only one of these genes is necessary to handle the normal metabolic demands, and individuals with one normal and one abnormal gene function and develop well. However, when each parent has one abnormal and one normal gene, on average one out of every four of their children will inherit the abnormal gene from each parent, and thus have a pair of abnormal genes. In such affected individuals, with a double dose of the abnormal gene, phenylalanine is not broken down normally and phenylalanine blood concentrations rise dramatically to levels severely toxic for the developing nervous system. Individuals with PKU develop severe retardation. By the age of six months, impaired mental development is evident and IQ falls from its initial normal levels of 100 to approximately 40 by the late teens. Most patients wind up in a variety of mental institutions, where they may account for as much as 1 percent of the total mentally retarded population.

As our understanding of the chemical basis of this devastating disease expanded, reliable and inexpensive blood tests were developed to detect the disorder in newborns. In the 1950s, effective therapy was developed based on diets free of the offending amino acid, phenylalanine. Individuals affected with PKU, when maintained on nonphenylalanine diets, will maintain normal intelligence and suffer none of the devastating consequences of their inherited abnormality. In fact, with long-term phenylalanine-free diets, some PKU patients who had already suffered severe loss of intelligence improve, though not nearly to normal IQ levels. Today all newborn children are screened before leaving the hospital for the presence of this genetic abnormality, and phenylalanine-free diets are widely available.

While there are other examples of the dramatic interdependence of genetics and environment, the PKU story underlines the essential fact that genetic endowment, by itself, does not necessarily determine the outcome in an individual.

CHAPTER 5
Prevention of Specific Diseases in Old Age

Hazzard, W., et al. (1990). Preventative gerontology: strategies for attenuation of the chronic disease of aging. *Principles of geriatric medicine and gerontology,* 2d ed., 167. New York: McGraw-Hill.

Rowe, J.W. (1990). Toward successful aging: limitation of the morbidity associated with "normal" aging. *Principles of geriatric medicine and gerontology,* 2d ed., 138. New York: McGraw-Hill.

Breast Cancer

Colditz, G.A., et al. (1995). The use of estrogens and progestins and the risk of breast cancer in postmenopausal women. *New England Journal of Medicine* 332(24):1589.

Prostate Cancer

Carter, B.H., et al. (1997). Recommended prostate-specific antigen testing intervals for the detection of curable prostate cancer. *Journal of the American Medical Association* 277:1456.

Catalona, W.J., et al. (1997). Prostate cancer detection in men with serum PSA concentrations of 2.6 to 4.0 ng/ml and benign prostate examination. Enhancement of specificity with free PSA measurements. *Journal of the American Medical Association* 277:1452.

Lung Cancer

Clark, L.C., et al. (1996). Effects of selenium supplementation for cancer prevention in patients with carcinoma of the skin. *Journal of the American Medical Association* 276:1957.

Colditz, G.A. (1996). Selenium and cancer prevention (editorial). *Journal of the American Medical Association* 276:1984.

Hennekens, C.H., et al. (1996). Lack of effect of long-term supplementation with beta-carotene on the incidence of malignant neoplasms and cardiovascular disease. *New England Journal of Medicine* 334:1145.

Omenn, G.S., et al. (1996). Effects of a combination of beta-carotene and vitamin A on lung cancer and cardiovascular disease. *New England Journal of Medicine* 334:1150.

Heart Disease

Barrett-Connor, E., et al. (1984). Ischemic heart disease risk factors after age 50. *Journal of Chronic Disease* 37:903.

Castelli, W.P., et al. (1989). Cardiovascular risk factors in the elderly. *American Journal of Cardiology* 63(suppl):12H.

Manson, J.E., et al. (1992). The primary prevention of myocardial infarction. *New England Journal of Medicine* 326:1406.

Marenberg, M.E., et al. (1994). Genetic susceptibility to death from coronary heart disease in a study of twins. *New England Journal of Medicine* 330(15):1041.

The Multiple Risk Factor Intervention Trial Research Group (1990). Mortality rates after 10.5 years for participants in the Multiple Risk Factor Intervention Trial: findings related to a prior hypotheses of the trial. *Journal of the American Medical Association* 263:1795.

Rich-Edwards, J.W., et al. (1995). The primary prevention of coronary heart disease in women. *New England Journal of Medicine* 332:1316.

Cholesterol

Anderson, K.M., et al. (1987). Cholesterol and mortality: 30 years of follow-up from the Framingham study. *Journal of the American Medical Association* 257:2176.

Aronow, W.S., et al. (1994). Correlation of serum lipids with the presence of coronary artery disease in 1,793 men and women aged less than 62 years. *American Journal of Cardiology* 73:702.

Benfante, R., et al. (1990). Is elevated serum cholesterol a risk factor for coronary health disease in the elderly? *Journal of the American Medical Association* 263:393.

Corti, M.C., et al. (1995). HDL cholesterol predicts coronary heart disease mortality in older persons. *Journal of the American Medical Association* 274:539.

Denke, M.A., et al. (1990). Hypercholesterolemia in elderly persons: resolving the treatment dilemma. *Annals of Internal Medicine* 112:780.

———. (1995). Cholesterol and coronary heart disease in older adults: no easy answers (editorial). *Journal of the American Medical Association* 274:575.

Grover, S.A., et al. (1992). The benefits of treating hyperlipidemia to prevent coronary heart disease. *Journal of the American Medical Association* 267:816.

Kalonek, S.D., et al. (1990). Treatment of hypercholesterolemia in the elderly (editorial). *Annals of Internal Medicine* 112:723.

Kronmal, R.A., et al. (1993). Total serum cholesterol levels and mortality risk as a function of age. *Archives of Internal Medicine* 153:1065.

Krumholz, H.M., et al. (1994). Lack of association between cholesterol and coronary heart disease mortality and morbidity and all-cause mortality in persons older than 70 years. *Journal of the American Medical Association* 272:1335.

Levine, G.N., et al. (1995). Cholesterol reduction in cardiovascular disease. *New England Journal of Medicine* 332:512.

Manninen, V., et al. (1988). Lipid alterations and decline in the incidence of coronary heart disease in the Helsinki study. *Journal of the American Medical Association* 260(5):641.

Manolio, T.A., et al. (1992). Cholesterol and heart disease in older persons and women: review of an NHBLI workshop. *Annals of Epidemiology* 2:161.

Oliver, M.F., et al. (September 5, 1984). WHO Cooperative Trial on primary prevention of ischaemic heart disease with clofibrate to lower serum cholesterol: final mortality follow-up. *Lancet.*

Schaefer, E.J., et al. (1994). Lipoprotein(a) levels and risk of coronary heart disease in men. *Journal of the American Medical Association* 271:999.

(1993). Summary of the second report of the national cholesterol education program (NCEP) expert panel on detection, evaluation, and treatment of high blood cholesterol in adults (Adult Treatment Panel II). *Journal of the American Medical Association* 269(23):3015.

(1984). The lipid research clinics coronary primary prevention trial results. I. Reduction in incidence of coronary heart disease. *Journal of the American Medical Association* 251:351.

Walsh, J.M.E., et al. (1995). Treatment of hyperlipidemia in women. *Journal of the American Medical Association* 274(14):1152.

Zimetbaum, P., et al. (1992). Plasma lipids and lipoproteins and the incidence of cardiovascular disease in the very elderly. *Arteriosclerosis and Thrombosis* 12:416.

Smoking

Hermanson, B., et al. (1988). Beneficial six-year outcome of smoking cessation in older men and women with coronary artery disease. *New England Journal of Medicine* 319:1365.

Higgins, M.W., et al. (1993). Smoking and lung function in elderly men and women. *Journal of the American Medical Association* 269:2741.

Hypertension

(1991). Prevention of stroke by antihypertensive drug treatment in older persons with isolated systolic hypertension. Final results of the Systolic Hypertension in the Elderly Program (SHEP). *Journal of the American Medical Association* 265:3255.

(1993). The fifth report of the Joint National Committee on detection, evaluation, and treatment of high blood pressure. *Archives of Internal Medicine* 153:154.

Syndrome X—Insulin Resistance and Diabetes Mellitus

Despres, J.P., et al. (1996). Hyperinsulinemia as an independent risk factor for ischemic heart disease. *New England Journal of Medicine* 334:952.

Donahue, R.P., et al. (1987). Post-challenge glucose concentration and coronary heart disease in men of Japanese ancestry: Honolulu heart program. *Diabetes* 36:189.

Elahi, D., et al. (1982). Effect of age and obesity on fasting levels of glucose, insulin, glucagon and growth hormone in man. *Journal of Gerontology* 37:485.

Foster, D.W. (1989). Insulin resistance—a secret killer (editorial). *New England Journal of Medicine* 320:733.

Gordon, T., et al. (1977). Diabetes, blood lipids, and the role of obesity in coronary heart disease risk for women: the Framingham study. *Annals of Internal Medicine* 87:393.

Katzel, L.I., et al. (1995). Effects of weight loss vs. aerobic exercise training on risk factors for coronary disease in healthy, obese, middle-aged, and older men. *Journal of the American Medical Association* 274:1915.

Kohrt, W.M., et al. (1990). Insulin resistance in aging is related to body composition. *Gerontologist* 30:38A.

Pyorala, K. (1979). Relationship of glucose tolerance and plasma insulin to the incidence of coronary heart disease: results of two population studies in Finland. *Diabetes Care* 2:131.

Zavaroni, I., et al. (1986). Effect of age and environmental factors on glucose tolerance and insulin secretion in a worker population. *Journal of the American Geriatrics Society* 34:271.

Postmenopausal Hormone Replacement Therapy

Col, N.F., et al. (1997). Patient-specific decisions about hormone replacement therapy in postmenopausal women. *Journal of the American Medical Association* 277:1140.

Grodstein, F., et al. (1997). Postmenopausal hormone therapy and mortality. *New England Journal of Medicine* 336:1769.

Nabulsi, A.A., et al. (1993). Association of hormone-replacement therapy with various cardiovascular risk factors in postmenopausal women. *New England Journal of Medicine* 328:1069.

Stampfer, M.J., et al. (1991). Postmenopausal estrogen therapy and cardiovascular disease. *New England Journal of Medicine* 325:756.

Aspirin

(1989). Final report on the aspirin component of the ongoing Physicians' Health Study. *New England Journal of Medicine* 321:129.

Manson, J.E., et al. (1991). A prospective study of aspirin use and primary prevention of cardiovascular disease in women. *Journal of the American Medical Association* 266:521.

Antioxidant Vitamins

Diaz, M.N., et al. (1997). Antioxidants and atherosclerotic heart disease. *New England Journal of Medicine* 337:408.

Jha, P., et al. (1995). The antioxidant vitamins and cardiovascular disease. *Annals of Internal Medicine* 123:860.

Rimm, E.B., et al. (1993). Vitamin E consumption and the risk of coronary heart disease in men. *New England Journal of Medicine* 328(20):1450.

Kushi, L.H., et al. (1996). Dietary antioxidant vitamins and death from coronary heart disease in postmenopausal women. *New England Journal of Medicine* 334:1156.

Homocysteine and Folic Acid

Boushey, C.J., et al. (1995). A quantitative assessment of plasma homocysteine as a risk factor for vascular disease. *Journal of the American Medical Association* 274:1049.

Nygard, O., et al. (1996). Total plasma homocysteine and cardiovascular risk profile. *Journal of the American Medical Association* 274:1526.

Riggs, K.M., et al. (1996). Relations of vitamin B-12, vitamin B-6, folate, and homocysteine to cognitive performance in the normative aging study. *American Journal for Clinical Nutrition* 63-306.

Zoler, M.L. (August 1, 1997). Folic acid intake inversely related to myocardial infarction risk. *Internal Medicine News.*

Stroke

Abbott, R.D., et al. (1987). Diabetes and the risk of stroke: the Honolulu heart program. *Journal of the American Medical Association* 257:949.

Boushey, C.J., et al. (1995). A quantitative assessment of plasma homocysteine as a risk factor for vascular disease: probable benefits of increasing folic acid intake. *Journal of the American Medical Association* 274:1049.

Graham, I.M., et al. (1997). Plasma homocysteine as a risk factor for vascular disease: the European concerted action project. *Journal of the American Medical Association* 277:1775.

Kawachi, I., et al. (1993). Smoking cessation and decreased risk of stroke in women. *Journal of the American Medical Association* 269:232.

Nygard, O., et al. (1995). Total plasma homocysteine and cardiovascular risk profile: the Hordaland homocysteine study. *Journal of the American Medical Association* 274:1526.

Osteoporosis

Birdwood, G. (1996). *Understanding osteoporosis and its treatment. A guide for physicians and their patients.* London: The Parthenon Publishing Group.

Prince, Richard L. (1997). Diet and the prevention of osteoporotic fractures. *New England Journal of Medicine* 337:701.

Hormone Replacement Therapy

Cauley, J.A., et al. (1995). Estrogen replacement therapy and fractures in older women. *Annals of Internal Medicine* 122(1):9.

Col, N.F., et al. (1997). Patient-specific decisions about hormone replacement therapy in postmenopausal women. *Journal of the American Medical Association* 277:1140.

Felson, D.T., et al. (1993). The effect of postmenopausal estrogen therapy on bone density in elderly women. *New England Journal of Medicine* 329(16):1141.

Grodstein, F., et al. (1997). Postmenopausal hormone therapy and mortality. *New England Journal of Medicine* 336:1769.

Kiel, D.P., et al. (1992). Smoking eliminates the protective effect of oral estrogens on the risk for hip fracture among women. *Annals of Internal Medicine* 116:716.

Lufkin, E.G., et al. (1992). Treatment of postmenopausal osteoporosis with transdermal estrogen. *Annals of Internal Medicine* 117(1):1.

Prince, R.L., et al. (1991). Prevention of postmenopausal osteoporosis. A comparative study of exercise, calcium supplementation, and hormone replacement therapy. *New England Journal of Medicine* 325(17):1189.

The Writing Group for the PEPI Trial. (1996). Effects of hormone therapy on bone mineral density. Results from the Postmenopausal Estrogen/Progestin Interventions (PEPI) Trial. *Journal of the American Medical Association* 276:1389.

Calcium and Vitamin D

Chopy, M.C., et al. (1992). Vitamin D3 and calcium to prevent hip fracture in elderly women. *New England Journal of Medicine.* 327(23):1637.

Dawson-Hughes, B., et al. (1997). Effect of calcium and vitamin D supplementation of bone density in men and women 65 years of age or older. *New England Journal of Medicine* 337:670.

Lips, P., et al. (1996). Vitamin D supplementation and fracture incidence in elderly persons. *Annals of Internal Medicine* 124:400.

Prince, R.L. (1997). Diet and the prevention of osteoporotic fractures. *New England Journal of Medicine* 337:701.

Reid, I.R., et al. (1993). Effect of calcium supplement on bone loss in postmenopausal women. *New England Journal of Medicine* 328:460.

Standing Committee on the Scientific Evaluation of Dietary Reference Intakes. Food and Nutrition Board, Institute of Medicine. (1997). Dietary reference intakes for calcium, phosphorus, magnesium, vitamin D, and fluoride. Washington, DC: National Academy Press.

Calcitonin

Azria, M., et al. (1995). 25 years of salmon calcitonin: from synthesis to therapeutic use. *Calcified Tissue International* 57(6):405.

Rico, H., et al. (1995). Total and regional bone mineral content and fracture rate in postmenopausal osteoporosis treated with salmon calcitonin: a prospective study. *Calcified Tissue International* 56:181.

Biphosphonates

Karpf, D.B., et al. (1997). Prevention of nonvertebral fractures by alendronate. A meta-analysis. *Journal of the American Medical Association* 277:1159.

Liberman, U.A., et al. (1995). Effect of alendronate on bone mineral density and the incidence of fractures in postmenopausal osteoporosis. *New England Journal of Medicine* 333(22):1437.

Fluoride

Pak, C.Y., et al. (1995). Treatment of postmenopausal osteoporosis with slow-release sodium fluoride. *Annals of Internal Medicine* 123(6):401.

Multi-Infarct Dementia

Skoog, I., et al. (1996). 15-year longitudinal study of blood pressure and dementia. *Lancet* 347:1141.

Alzheimer's Disease

Hormone Replacement

Birge, S.J. (1996). Is there a role for estrogen replacement therapy in the prevention and treatment of dementia? *Journal of the American Geriatrics Society* 44:865.

Tang, M.X., et al. (1996). Effect of oestrogen during menopause on risk and age at onset of Alzheimer's disease. *Lancet* 348:429.

Col, N.F., et al. (1997). Patient-specific decisions about hormone replacement therapy in postmenopausal women. *Journal of the American Medical Association* 277:1140.

Grodstein, F., et al. (1997). Postmenopausal hormone therapy and mortality. *New England Journal of Medicine* 336:1769.

Nonsteroidal Anti-inflammatory Drugs (NSAIDs)

Rozzini, R., et al. (1996). Protective effect of chronic NSAID use on cognitive decline in older persons. *Journal of the American Geriatrics Society* 44:1025.

Vitamin Supplementation

Boushey, C.J., et al. (1995). A quantitative assessment of plasma homocysteine as a risk factor for vascular disease: probable benefits of increasing folic acid intakes. *Journal of the American Medical Association* 274:1049.

Graham, I.M., et al. (1997). Plasma homocysteine as a risk factor for vascular disease: the European concerted action project. *Journal of the American Medical Association* 277:1775.

Naurath, H., et al. (1995). Effects of vitamin B12, folate, and vitamin B6 supplements in elderly people with normal serum vitamin levels. *Lancet* 346:85.

Nygard, O., et al. (1995). Total plasma homocysteine and cardiovascular risk profile: the Hordaland homocysteine study. *Journal of the American Medical Association* 274:1526.

Riggs, K.M., et al. (1996). Relations of vitamin B12, vitamin B6, folate, and homocysteine to cognitive performance in the normative aging study. *American Journal of Clinical Nutrition* 63:306.

CHAPTER 6

What Happens to the Body as We Age

Buskirk, E.R., et al. (1987). Age and aerobic power: the rate of change in men and women. *Federation Proceedings* 46:1824.

Kohrt, W.M., et al. (1991). Effects of gender, age and fitness level on response of Vo₂max to training in 60- to 70-year-olds. *Journal of Applied Physiology* 71:2004.

Raven, P.B., et al. (1980). The effect of aging on the cardiovascular response to dynamic and static exercise. In Weisfeldt, M.L., ed., *The aging heart*, 269. New York: Raven Press.

Exercise for Older People

U.S. Department of Health and Human Services. (1996). Physical activity and health: a report of the Surgeon General. Atlanta, GA: U.S. Department of Health and Human Services, Centers for Disease Control and Prevention, National Center for Chronic Disease Prevention and Health Promotion.

Sticht, J.P., et al. (1995). Weight control and exercise: cardinal features of successful preventative gerontology (editorial). *Journal of the American Medical Association* 274:1964.

Aerobic Exercise

Brown, M., et al. (1991). Effects of low-intensity exercise program on selected physical performance characteristics of 60- to 71-year olds. *Aging* 3:129.

Buchner, D.M., et al. (1992). Effects of physical activity on health status in older adults II: intervention studies. *Annual Review of Public Health* 13:469.

Evans, W.J. (1995). Effects of exercise on body composition and functional capacity of the elderly. *Journal of Gerontology* 50A:147.

Fabre, C., et al. (1997). Effectiveness of individualized aerobic training at the ventilatory threshold in the elderly. *Journal of Perontology: Biological Sciences* 52A(5), B260.

Holloszy, J.O., et al. (1986). Effects of exercise on glucose tolerance and insulin resistance. *Acta Medica Scandinavia* (suppl.) 711:55.

Meredith, C.N., et al. (1989). Peripheral effects of endurance training in young and old subjects. *Journal of Applied Physiology* 66:2844.

Morey, M.C., et al. (1991). Two-year trends in physical performance following supervised exercise among community-dwelling older veterans. *Journal of the American Geriatrics Society* 39:549.

Rogers, M.A., et al. (1993). Changes in skeletal muscle with aging: Effects of exercise training. *Exercise and Sport Science Reviews* 21:65.

Seals, D.R., et al. (1984b). Endurance training in older men and women: cardiovascular responses to exercise. *Journal of Applied Physiology* (Respirat Environ Exer Physiol) 57:1024.

Weight Training

Ades, P.A., et al. (1996). Weight training improves walking endurance in healthy elderly persons. *Annals of Internal Medicine* 124.

Campbell, W.W., et al. (1995). Effects of resistance training and dietary protein intake on protein metabolism in older adults. *American Journal of Physiology* 268:E1143.

Fiatarone, M.A., et al. (1990). High-intensity strength training in nonagenarians. *Journal of the American Medical Association* 263:3029.

———. (1994). Exercise training and nutritional supplementation for physical frailty in very elderly people. *New England Journal of Medicine* 330:1769.

Frontera, W.R., et al. (1988). Strength conditioning in older men: skeletal muscle hypertrophy and improved function. *Journal of Applied Physiology* 64:1038.

———. (1990). Strength training and determinants of Vo_2max in older men. *Journal of Applied Physiology* 68:329.

Judge, J.O., et al. (1994). Effects of resistive and balance exercises on isokinetic strength in older persons. *Journal of the American Geriatric Society* 42:937.

McCartney, N. (1996). A longitudinal trial of weight training in the elderly: continued improvements in year 2. *Journal of Gerontology* 51A:B425.

Pratley, R., et al. (1994). Strength training increases resting metabolic rate and norepinephrine levels in healthy 50- to 65-year-old men. *Journal of Applied Physiology* 76:133.

Singh, N.A., et al. (1997). A randomized controlled trial of progressive resistance training in depressed elders. *Journal of Gerontology* 52(1):M27.

Risks of Exercise

Harris, S.S., et al. (1989). Physical activity counseling for healthy adults as a primary preventive intervention in the clinical setting. *Journal of the American Medical Association* 261:3590.

Lai, J-S., et al. (1995). Two-year trends in cardiorespiratory function among older Tai Chi Chuan practitioners and sedentary subjects. *Journal of American Geriatrics Society* 43:1222.

Nelson, M.E. (1997). *Strong women stay young.* New York: Bantam Books.

Pollack, M.L., et al. (1991). Injuries and adherence to walk/jog and resistance training programs in the elderly. *Medicine and Science in Sports and Exercise* 23:1194.

Physical Fitness and the Risk of Specific Diseases

Blair, S.N., et al. (1992). How much physical activity is good for health? *Annual Review of Public Health* 13:99.

———. (1995). Changes in physical fitness and all-cause mortality: A prospective study of healthy and unhealthy men. *Journal of the American Medical Association* 273:1093.

———. (1996). Influences of cardiorespiratory fitness and other precursors on cardiovascular disease and all-cause mortality in men and women. *Journal of the American Medical Association* 276:205.

Chang-Claude, J., et al. (1993). Dietary and lifestyle determinants of mortality among German vegetarians. *International Journal of Epidemiology* 22:228.

Kaplan, G.A., et al. (1987). Mortality among the elderly in the Alameda County Study: behavioral and demographic risk factors. *American Journal of Public Health* 77:307.

Kushi, L.H., et al. (1997). Physical activity and mortality in post-menopausal women. *Journal of the American Medical Association* 277:1287.

Leon, A.S., et al. (1991). Physical activity and 10.5 year mortality in the Multiple Risk Factor Intervention Trial (MRFIT). *International Journal of Epidemiology* 20:690.

Lindsted, K.D., et al. (1991). Self-report of physical activity and patterns of mortality in Seventh-day Adventist men. *Journal of Clinical Epidemiology* 44:355.

Paffenbarger, Jr., R.S., et al. (1993). The association of changes in physical-activity level and other lifestyle characteristics with mortality among men. *New England Journal of Medicine* 328:538.

Thune, I., et al. (1997). Physical activity and the risk of breast cancer. *New England Journal of Medicine* 336:1269.

Coronary Heart Disease

Berlin, J.A., et al. (1990). A meta-analysis of physical activity in the prevention of coronary heart disease. *American Journal of Epidemiology* 132:612.

Folsom, A.R., et al. (1985). Leisure-time physical activity and its relationship to coronary risk factors in a population-based sample: the Minnesota heart survey. *American Journal of Epidemiology* 121:570.

Katzel, L.I., et al. (1995). Effects of weight loss vs. aerobic exercise training on risk factors for coronary disease in healthy, obese, middle-aged, and older men. *Journal of the American Medical Association* 274:1915.

Leon, A.S., et al. (1987). Leisure-time physical activity levels and risk of coronary heart disease and death. *Journal of the American Medical Association* 258:2388.

Slattery, M.L., et al. (1988). Physical fitness and cardiovascular disease mortality: the U.S. railroad study. *American Journal of Epidemiology* 127:571.

―――. (1989). Leisure-time physical activity and coronary heart disease death: the U.S. railroad study. *Circulation* 79:304.

High Blood Pressure

Arroll, B., et al. (1992). Does physical activity lower blood pressure? A critical review of the clinical trials. *Journal of Clinical Epidemiology* 45:419.

Blair, S.N., et al. (1984). Physical fitness and incidence of hypertension in healthy normotensive men and women. *Journal of the American Medical Association* 252:487.

Folsom, A.R., et al. (1990). Incidence of hypertension and stroke in relation to body fat distribution and other risk factors in older women. *Stroke* 21:701.

Hagberg, J.M., et al. (1989). Effect of exercise training in 60- to 69-year-old persons with essential hypertension. *American Journal of Cardiology* 64:348.

Kelley, G., et al. (1994). Antihypertensive effects of aerobic exercise: a brief meta-analytic review of randomized controlled trials. *American Journal of Hypertension* 7:115.

Matsusaki, M., et al. (1992). Influence of workload on the antihypertensive effect of exercise. *Clinical Experimental Pharmacology and Physiology* 19:471.

Diabetes

Miller, J.P., et al. (1994). Strength training increases insulin action in healthy 50- to 65-year-old men. *Journal of Applied Physiology* 77:1122.

Rogers, M.A., et al. (1993). Changes in skeletal muscle with aging: effects of exercise training. *Exercise and Sport Science Reviews* 21:65.

Ryan, A.S., et al. (1996). Resistive training increases insulin action in postmenopausal women. *Journal of Gerontology: Biological Science* 51A:M199.

Seals, D.R., et al. (1984). Effects of endurance training on glucose tolerance and plasma lipid levels in older men and women. *Journal of the American Medical Association* 252:654.

Arthritis

Allegrante, J.P., et al. (1993). A walking education program for patients with osteoarthritis of the knee: theory and intervention strategies. *Health Education Quarterly* 20:63.

Ettinger, W.H., Jr., et al. (1994). Physical disability from knee osteoarthritis: the role of exercise as an intervention. *Medicine and Science in Sports and Exercise* 26:1435.

Fisher, N.M., et al. (1991). Muscle rehabilitation: its effect on muscular and functional performance of patients with knee osteoarthritis. *Archives of Physical Medicine and Rehabilitation* 72:367.

———. (1994). Quantitative evaluation of a home exercise program on muscle and functional capacity of patients with osteoarthritis. *American Journal of Physical Medical Rehabilitation* 75:792.

Minor, M.A., et al. (1989). Efficacy of physical conditioning exercise in patients with rheumatoid arthritis and osteoarthritis. *Arthritis Rheum* 32:1396.

———. (1993). Exercise maintenance of persons with arthritis after participation in a class experience. *Health Education Quarterly* 20:83.

Osteoporosis

Kohrt, W.M., et al. (1995). Additive effects of weight-bearing exercise and estrogen on bone mineral density in older women. *Journal of Bone and Mineral Research* 10:1303.

Nelson, M.E., et al. (1994). Positive effects of high-intensity strength training on multiple risk factors for osteoporotic fractures. *Journal of the American Medical Association* 272:1909.

Prince, R.L. (1997). Diet and the prevention of osteoporotic fractures. *New England Journal of Medicine* 337:701.

Prince, R.L., et al. (1991). Prevention of postmenopausal osteoporosis: a comparative study of exercise, calcium supplementation, and hormone-replacement therapy. *New England Journal of Medicine* 325:1189.

Standing Committee on the Scientific Evaluation of Dietary Reference Intakes. Food and Nutrition Board, Institute of Medicine. (1997). Dietary reference intakes for calcium, phosphorus, magnesium, vitamin D, and fluoride. Washington, DC: National Academy Press.

Testosterone

Lamberts, S.W.J., et al. (1997). The endocrinology of aging. *Science* 278:419.

Falls and Balance

Crilly, R.G., et al. (1989). Effect of exercise on postural sway in the elderly. *Gerontology* 35:137.

Era, P., et al. (1985). Postural sway during standing and unexpected disturbance of balance in random samples of men of different ages. *Journal of Gerontology* 40:287.

Judge, J.O., et al. (1993). Balance improvements in older women: effects of exercise training. *Physical Therapy* 73:254.

————. (1993). Exercise to improve gait velocity in older persons. *Archives of Physical Medicine and Rehabilitation* 74:400.

Ledin, T., et al. (1991). Effects of balance training in elderly evaluated by clinical tests and dynamic posturography. *Journal of Vestibular Research* 1:129.

Lord, S.R., et al. (1995). The effect of exercise on balance and related factors in older women: a randomized control trial. *Journal of the American Geriatrics Society* 43:1198.

Province, M.A., et al. (1995). The effects of exercise on falls in elderly patients: a preplanned meta-analysis of the FICSIT trials. *Journal of the American Medical Association* 273:1341.

Reinsch, S., et al. (1992). Attempts to prevent falls and injury: a prospective community study. *Gerontologist* 32:450.

Tinetti, M.E., et al. (1994). A multifactorial intervention to reduce the risk of falling among elderly people living in the community. *New England Journal of Medicine* 331:821.

Topp, R., et al. (1993). The effect of a 12-week dynamic resistance strength training program on gait velocity and balance in older adults. *Gerontologist* 33:501.

Wolf, S.L., et al. (1993). The Atlanta FICSIT study: two exercise interventions to reduce frailty in elders. *Journal of the American Geriatrics Society* 41:329.

————. (1996). Reducing frailty and falls in older persons: an investigation of Tai Chi and computerized balance training. *Journal of the American Geriatrics Society* 44:489.

Wolfson, L., et al. (1996). Balance and strength training in older adults: intervention gains and Tai Chi maintenance. *Journal of the American Geriatrics Society* 44:498.

Nutrition in Old Age

Meydani, S., et al. (1991). Elderly adults. *American Journal of Clinical Nutrition* 53:1275.

Morley, J.E., et al. (1990). *Geriatric nutrition, a comprehensive review*, 45. New York: Raven Press.

Recommended dietary allowances. 10th edition (1989). Washington, DC: National Academy Press.

Reichel, W. (1995). *Care of the elderly: clinical aspects of aging.* 4th ed., 229. Baltimore: Williams and Wilkins.

Rimm, E.B., et al. (1996). Vegetable, fruit, and cereal fiber intake and risk of coronary heart disease among men. *Journal of the American Medical Association* 257:447.

Standing Committee on the Scientific Evaluation of Dietary Reference Intakes. Food and Nutrition Board, Institute of Medicine. (1997). Dietary reference intakes for calcium, phosphorus, magnesium, vitamin D, and fluoride. Washington, DC: National Academy Press.

Wellman, N.S. (March 21, 1994). Dietary guidance and nutrient requirements of the elderly. *Primary Care* 1.

Vitamins

Boushey, C.J., et al. (1995). A quantitative assessment of plasma homocysteine as a risk factor for vascular disease. *Journal of the American Medical Association* 274:1049.

Lindenbaum, J., et al. (1988). Neuropsychiatric disorders caused by cobalamin deficiency in the absence of anemia or macrocytosis. *New England Journal of Medicine* 318:1720.

Nygard, O., et al. (1995). Total plasma homocysteine and cardiovascular risk profile. *Journal of the American Medical Association* 274:1526.

Riggs, K.M., et al. (1996). Relations of vitamin B12, vitamin B6, folate, and homocysteine to cognitive performance in the normative aging study. *American Journal of Clinical Nutrition* 63:306.

Russel, R.M., et al. (1986). Folic acid metabolism in atrophic gastritis. *Gastroenterology* 91:1476–82.

Antioxidants

The Alpha-Tocopherol, Beta-Carotene Cancer Prevention Study Group. (1994). The effect of Vitamin E and beta-carotene on the incidence of lung cancer and other cancer in male smokers. *New England Journal of Medicine* 330:1029.

Chandra, R.K. (1997). Graying of the immune system: can nutrient supplements improve immunity in the elderly? (editorial). *Journal of the American Medical Association* 277:1396.

Clark, L.C., et al. (1996). Effects of selenium supplementation for cancer prevention in patients with carcinoma of the skin. *Journal of the American Medical Association* 276:1957.

Graham, et al. (December 25, 1996). Selenium and cancer prevention: promising results indicate further trials required (editorial). *Journal of the American Medical Association* 276:24.

Hennekens, C.H., et al. (1996). Lack of effect of long-term supplementation with beta-carotene on the incidence of malignant neoplasms and cardiovascular disease. *New England Journal of Medicine* 334:1145.

Jha, P., et al. (1995). The antioxidant vitamins and cardiovascular disease: a critical review of epidemiologic and clinical data. *Annals of Internal Medicine* 123:860.

Losonczy, K.G., et al. (1996). Vitamin E and vitamin C supplement use and risk of all-cause and coronary heart disease mortality in older persons: the established populations for epidemiologic studies of the elderly. *American Journal of Clinical Nutrition* 64:190.

Meydani, S.N., et al. (1997). Vitamin E supplementation and in vivo immune response in healthy elderly subjects. *Journal of the American Medical Association* 277:1380.

Rimm, E.B., et al. (1993). Vitamin E consumption and the risk of coronary heart disease in men. *New England Journal of Medicine* 328:1450.

Stampfer, et al. (1993). Vitamin E consumption and the risk of coronary disease in women. *New England Journal of Medicine.* 328:1444.

Stephens, N.G., et al. (1996). Randomized controlled trial of vitamin E in patients with coronary disease: Cambridge Heart Antioxidant Study (CHAOS). *Lancet* 347:781.

Wood, R.J., et al. (1995). Mineral requirement of elderly people. *American Journal of Clinical Nutrition* 62:493.

CHAPTER 7

Berkman, L., et al. (1993). High, usual and impaired functioning in community-dwelling elderly: MacArthur successful aging field studies. *Clinical Epidemiology* 46(10):1129.

Bruce, M., et al. (1994). The impact of depressive symptomatology on physical disability: MacArthur studies of successful aging. *American Journal of Public Health* 84(11):1796.

Guralnik, J., et al. (1994). Validation and use of performance measures of functioning in a non-disabled older population: MacArthur studies of successful aging. *AGING: Clinical and Experimental Research* 6(6):410.

Seeman, T., et al. (1994). Predicting changes in physical functioning in a high-functioning elderly cohort: MacArthur studies of successful aging. *Journal of Gerontology* 49:M97.

———. (1995). Behavioral and psychosocial predictors of physical performance: MacArthur studies of successful aging. *Journal of Gerontology* 50A:M177.

CHAPTER 8

Harris, L., et al. (1981). *Aging in the eighties: America in transition.* Washington, DC: National Council on Aging.

Commonwealth Fund. (1993). *The untapped resource.* New York, NY.

How Worried Should Older People Be About Decreasing Mental Function?

Institute for Social Research. (1997). *Overview of the AHEAD study.* Ann Arbor, MI: Institute for Social Research.

Khachaturian, Z.S., and Radebaugh, T.S. (1997). *Alzheimer's disease: diagnosis, treatment, and care.* Boca Raton, FL: CRC Press.

Manton, K., and Stallard, E. (1984). *Recent trends in mortality analysis.* Orlando, FL: Academic Press.

———. (1996). Longevity in the United States: age and sex-specific evidence on life-span limits from mortality patterns 1960–1990. *Journal of Gerontology: Biological Sciences* 51A: 362.

National Institute on Aging. (August 1995). *Alzheimer's disease and related dementias: biomedical update.* Washington, DC: Department of Health and Human Services.

Are Cognitive Losses an Inevitable Part of Aging?

Allen, P.A., et al. (1997). Age differences in mental multiplication: evidence for peripheral but not central decrements. *Journal of Gerontology* 52B(2), 81.

Cerella, J. (1990). Aging and information-processing rate. In Birren, J.E., and Schaie, K.W., eds., *Handbook of the psychology of aging* 3:201. San Diego: Academic.

Chipuer, H.M., et al. (1990). LISREL modeling: genetic and environmental influences on IQ revisited. *Intelligence* 14:11.

Herzog, A.R., and Rodgers, W.L. (1989). Age differences in memory performance and memory ratings as measured in a sample survey. *Psychology and Aging* 4(2):173.

Hultsch, D.F., and Dixon, R.A. (1990). Learning and memory in aging. In Birren, J.E., and Schaie, K.W., eds., *Handbook of the psychology of aging* 3:258. San Diego: Academic.

Lehman, H.C. (1953). *Age and achievement.* Princeton, NJ: Princeton University Press.

McDowd, J.M., and Birren, J.E. (1990). Aging and attentional process. In Birren, J.E., and Schaie, K.W., eds., *Handbook of the psychology of aging* 3:222. San Diego: Academic.

Morrison, J.H. and Hob, P.R. (1977). Life and death of neurons in the aging brain. *Science* 278:412.

Schaie, K.W. (1990). Optimization of cognitive functioning: predictions based on cohort-sequential and longitudinal data. In Baltes, P.B., and Baltes, M.M., eds., *Successful aging: perspectives from the behavioral sciences.* Cambridge, UK: Cambridge University Press.

Wickelgren, I. (1997). Estrogen stakes claim to cognition. *Science* 276:675.

Can Decreases in Mental Function Be Prevented?

Genetic Factors in Cognitive Function

Loehlin, J.C. (1989). Partitioning environmental and genetic contributions to behavioral development. *American Psychologist* 44:1285.

McClearn, G.E., et al. (1997). Substantial genetic influence on cognitive abilities in twins 80+ years old. *Science* 276:1560.

Enduring Properties of the Person

Albert, M.S., et al. (1995). Predictors of cognitive change in older persons: MacArthur studies of successful aging. *Psychology and Aging* 10(4):578.

Bandura, A. (1997). *Self-efficacy: the exercise of control.* New York: Freeman.

Brown, I., Jr., and Inouye, D.K. (1978). Learned helplessness through modeling. *Journal of Personality and Social Psychology* 36:900.

Collins, J.L. (1982). *Self-efficacy and ability in achievement behavior.* Paper presented at the annual meeting of the American Educational Research Association.

Cook, N.R., et al. (1989). Peak expiratory flow rate and 5- to 6-year mortality in an elderly population. *American Journal of Epidemiology* 130:66.

Gist, M.E., et al. (1989). Effects of alternative training methods on self-efficacy and performance in computer software training. *Journal of Applied Psychology* 74:884.

Lachman, M.E., et al. (1995). Assessing memory control beliefs: the memory controllability inventory. *Aging and Cognition* 2:67.

Neeper, S.A., et al. (1995). Exercise and brain neurotrophins. *Nature* 373:109.

Seligman, M.E.P. (1975). *Helplessness: on depression, development, and death.* San Francisco: Freeman.

The concept of learned helplessness was first developed and demonstrated experimentally by Martin E.P. Seligman. He showed that dogs that had re-peatedly been restrained from avoiding an unpleasant stimulus (electric shock) continued to endure it even after the restraints were removed. The repeated experience of physical helplessness had taught them that attempts to escape were useless. This "learning" persisted even after the conditions that produced it were no longer in force.

Turner, N., et al. (1997). Exercise training reverses the age-related decline in tyrosine hudroxylase expression in rat hypothalamus. *Journal of Gerontology: Biological Sciences* 52A(5):B255.

Environmental Influences on Cognitive Function

Kohn, M.L., and Schooler, C. (1983). *Work and personality: an inquiry into the impact of social stratification.* Norwood, NJ: Ablex.

Miller, J., et al. (1979). Women and work: The psychological effects of occupa-tional conditions. *American Journal of Sociology* 85:66.

————. (1985). Continuity of learning-generalization throughout the life span. *American Journal of Sociology* 91:593.

Miller, K.A., et al. (1986). Educational self-direction and cognitive functioning of students. *Social Forces* 63:923.

Naoi, A., and Schooler, C. (1986). Occupational conditions and psychological functioning in Japan. *American Journal of Sociology* 90:372.

Schooler, C., et al. (1983). Housework as work. In Kohn, M.L., and Schooler, C., eds., *Work and personality: An inquiry into the impact of social stratification,* 242. Norwood, NJ: Ablex.

Schooler, C., and Schaie, K.W. (1987). *Cognitive functioning and social structure over the life course.* Norwood, NJ: Ablex.

Schooler, C. (1990). Psychosocial factors and effective cognitive functioning in adulthood. In Birren, J.E., and Schaie, K.W., eds., *Handbook of the psychology of aging* 3:347. San Diego: Academic.

Can Older People Increase Any of Their Mental Abilities?

Avorn, J., and Langer, E.J. (1982). Induced disability in nursing home patients: a controlled trial. *Journal of the American Geriatric Society* 30(6):397.

Berry, J.M. (1996). A self-efficacy model of memory function in adulthood. Submitted for publication.

Diaz, M.N., Frei, B., et al. (1997). Anti-oxidants and atherosclerotic heart disease. *New England Journal of Medicine* 337:408.

Kahn, R.L., and Antonucci, T.C. (1981). Convoys of social support: a life-course approach. In Kiesler, S.B., et al., eds., *Aging: social change*, 383. New York: Academic Press.

Kliegl, R., et al. (1989). Testing the limits and the study of adult age differences in cognitive plasticity of a mnemonic skill. *Developmental Psychology* 25:247.

Schaie, K.W., and Willis, S.L. (1986). Can adult intellectual decline be reversed? *Developmental Psychology* 22:223.

Wickelgren, I. (1997). Estrogen stakes claim to cognition. *Science* 276:675.

Wisdom in Old Age: Beyond the Imitation of Youth

Baltes, P.B., et al. (1992). Wisdom and successful aging. In Sonderegger T.B., ed., *Nebraska symposium on motivation* 39:123. Lincoln, NB: University of Nebraska Press.

Sternberg, R.J., ed. (1990). *Wisdom: its nature, origins, and development*. Cambridge, UK: Cambridge University Press.

CHAPTER 9

DHEA

Barrett-Connor, E., et al. (1986). A prospective study of DHEA-S, mortality, and cardiovascular disease. *New England Journal of Medicine* 315:1519.

Cassor, P., et al. (1993). Oral DHEA in physiologic doses modulates immune function in postmenopausal women. *American Journal of Obstetrics and Gynecology* 169:1536.

Khorram, O., et al. (1997). Activation of immune function by dehydroepiandrosterone (DHEA) in age-advanced men. *Journal of Gerontology* 52A:M1.

The Medical Letter (October 1996). 38 (985):91.

Morales, A.F., et al. (1994). Effects of replacement doses of DHEA in men and women of advancing age. *Journal of Clinical Endocrinology Metabolism* 78:1360.

Orentreich, N., et al. (1992). Long-term longitudinal measurements of plasma DHEA-S in normal men. *Journal of Clinical Endocrinology Metabolism* 75:1002.

Melatonin

Brzezinski, A. (1997). Melatonin in humans. *New England Journal of Medicine* 336:186.

Dollins, A.B., et al. (1994). Effect of inducing nocturnal serum melatonin concentrations in daytime on sleep, mood, body temperature, and performance. *Proceedings of National Academy of Science* 91:1824.

Garfinkel, D., et al. (1995). Improvement of sleep quality in elderly people by controlled-release melatonin. *Lancet* 346:541.

The Medical Letter (November 1995). 37(962):111.

Petrie, K., et al. (1989). Effect of melatonin on jet lag after long-haul flights. *British Medical Journal* 28:705.

Human Growth Hormone

Butterfield, G.E., et al. (1996). Effect of rhGH and rhIGF-I treatment on protein utilization in elderly women. *American Journal of Physiology* E94.

(October 1996). Can hormones reverse aging? NIA, National Institutes of Health. *The Public Information Office*, 1.

Corpoas, E., et al. (1993). Human growth hormone and human aging. *Endocrine Reviews* 14(1):20.

Gambert, S.R., et al. (June 1995). Endocrinology and metabolism clinics of North America. *Endocrine Aspects of Aging* 23(2):221.

Holloway, L., et al. (1994). Effects of recombinant human growth hormone on metabolic indices, body composition, and bone turnover in healthy elderly women. *Journal of Clinical Endocrinology Metabolism* 79:470.

Papadakis, M.A., et al. (1996). Growth hormone replacement in healthy older men improves body composition but not functional ability. *Annals of Internal Medicine* 124:708.

Rudman, D., et al. (1990). Effects of human growth hormone in men over 60 years old. *New England Journal of Medicine* 323:1.

———. (1991). Effects of human growth hormone on body composition in elderly men. *Hormone Research* 36 (suppl 1):73.

Anti-aging Skin Treatments

Gardner, S.S., et al. (1990). Clinical features of photodamage and treatment with topical tretinoin. *Journal of Dermatology and Surgical Oncology* 16:925.

Goldfarb, M.T., et al. (1990). Topical tretinoin: its use in daily practice to reverse photoaging. *British Journal of Dermatology* 35:87.

Griffiths, C.E.M., et al. (1995). Two concentrations of topical tretinoin (retinoic acid) cause similar improvement of photoaging but different degrees of irritation. *Archives of Dermatology* 131:1037.

Humphreys, T.R., et al. (1996). Treatment of photodamaged skin with trichloroacetic acid and topical tretinoin. *Journal of the American Academy of Dermatology* 34:638.

Lyden, J.J., et al. (1989). Treatment of photodamaged facial skin with topical tretinoin. *Journal of the American Academy of Dermatology* 21:638.

Moy, L.S., et al. (1993). Glycolic acid peels for the treatment of wrinkles and photoaging. *Journal of Dermatology and Surgical Oncology* 19:243.

CHAPTER 10

Forster, E.M. (1911). *Howard's end.* New York and London: Putnam.

The Meaning of Connectedness

Spitz, R. (1971). The adaptive viewpoint: its role in autism and child psychiatry. *Journal of Autism and Childhood Schizophrenia* 1(3):239.

Spitz, working within a psychoanalytic framework, was an early researcher on the positive effects of nurturant behavior in infancy and the damaging effects of its absence, even when physical needs for food and clothing were being met.

His work is part of an immense and still growing research literature on the developmental importance of touching, caressing, and other forms of interaction between infants and their caregivers.

Lane, H. (1976). *The wild boy of Aveyron.* Cambridge: Harvard University Press.

Lane's book is an intensive study of an already famous case. For earlier discussion, see:

Gayral L., et al. (1972). The first observations in the wild-boy of Lacaune (called "Victor" or "the wild-boy of Aveyron"): new documents. *Annales Medico-Psychologiques* 2(4):465.

For reviews of such cases, see:

McNeil, M.C., et al. (1984). Feral and isolated children: historical review and analysis. *Education and Training of the Mentally Retarded* 19(1):70.

Also see:

Favazza, A.R. (1977). Feral and isolated children. *British Journal of Medical Psychology* 50(1):105.

Goldberger, L. (1970). In the absence of stimuli. *Science* 168:709.

(July 26, 1996). Gene may be clue to nature of nurturing. *New York Times.*

Connectedness and Survival

Durkheim, E. (1951). *Suicide* (trans.). Glencoe, IL: Free Press.

Emile Durkheim, the famous French social philosopher and researcher, is considered one of the founders of sociology as a distinct discipline. His many writings deal with such fundamental questions as the division of labor in society, the societal role of religion, and the methods of sociological research. His study of suicide, first published in French in 1897 (*Le suicide: étude de sociologie.* Paris: F. Alcan), is important both for its substantive linking of social isolation (anomie) to suicide and for its use of quantitative data to test a sociological hypothesis. The English translation of *Le suicide* (1951. *Suicide: A study in sociology.* Glencoe, Illinois: Free Press) remains required reading for students of sociology.

Berkman, L.S., and Syme, S.L. (1979). Social networks, host resistance, and mortality: a nine year follow-up study of Alameda County residents. *American Journal of Epidemiology* 109:186.

The authors conducted a survey in northern California that included an "index of social integration" based on four measures: marital status, contacts with family and friends, church membership, and membership in other organized groups. They then recorded the deaths among survey respondents during the next nine years in order to determine the statistical relationship between their social integration index and the probability of death. The result made the study famous: social integration was a significant predictor of longevity; people who lacked social ties died earlier.

House, J.S., et al. (July 29, 1988). Social relationships and health. *Science* 241: 540.

At least four other studies, two in the United States and two in Scandinavia, have replicated and enlarged upon the Alameda County finding. House, Landis, and Umberson (1988) summarize and compare the results of these five studies. There are differences among them. For example, the Evans County (Georgia) study showed the expected relationship between social support and longevity for white men, but the relationship was not significant among black men. In studies that included comparisons between men and women, the effect of social support was stronger for men than for women. There is some evidence that the positive effect of social relationships comes mainly from the difference between low and average connectedness and tends to taper off thereafter.

The main point holds, however; people whose connections with others are relatively strong, through family, friends, and organizational memberships, live longer. For people whose relationships to others are relatively few and weak, the risk of death, irrespective of age, is two to four times as great.

The Gothenberg (Sweden) study is particularly important for gerontology because it included two groups of elderly men, one set born in 1913 and the other in 1923. As the Gothenberg data show, we do not outgrow our need for others; the life-giving effect of close relations holds throughout the life course.

Social Support: The Essential Ingredient

Cobb, S. (1976). Social support as a moderator of life stress. *Psychosomatic Medicine* 38(5):300.

Cobb, a physician and epidemiologist, proposed this definition (love, care, esteem, mutual obligation) in a wide-ranging review of previous research. Cassel, working independently, published a similar review during the same year. Both researchers realized that no one of the studies they cited demonstrated a cause-and-effect relationship between social support and health, since almost all of them were cross-sectional in design and were based on self-report. Both Cobb and Cassel felt, however, that the number of such studies, the variety of settings, the wide range of health outcomes, and the convergence of research results argued strongly in favor of the key proposition that social support is health protective.

Other researchers were persuaded, and the years following the Cobb and Cassel articles saw a flood of research on social support. Most of it has confirmed their basic findings and some of it has begun to answer questions that their findings suggested: What are the pathways or mechanisms by which social support protects people against stress and enhances their health? And how do the general findings on social support apply to specific situations and groups, especially older men and women?

Antonucci, T.C., et al. (1989). Psychosocial factors and the response to cancer symptoms. In Yancik, R., and Yates, J.W., eds., *Cancer in the elderly: approaches to early detection and treatment,* 40. New York: Springer.

Berkman, L.F. (1983). *Social networks and social support.* Paper presented at the NHLBI Workshop, Galveston, TX.

Cassel, J. (1976). The contribution of the social environment to host resistance. *American Journal of Epidemiology* 104:107.

Kahn, R.L. (1979). Aging and social support. In Riley, M.W., ed., *Aging from birth to death*. Boulder, CO: Westview.

What Does Social Support Consist Of?

The articles by Kahn, Antonucci, and their colleagues are based on data from a national survey, Social Supports of the Elderly, conducted by the Survey Research Center (University of Michigan) and supported by the National Institute on Aging. The concept of the convoy was developed in the course of this work, as was the hierarchical technique for mapping the pattern of support provided by convoy members.

The findings on reciprocity (Ingersoll-Dayton and Antonucci) and on veridicality (Antonucci and Israel) stem from a unique feature of this survey: Interviews were conducted with convoy members to determine the extent of agreement about the nature and amount of support provided. It then became possible to see whether network members reported providing support to people who had named them as sources of support. Results of this analysis were summarized as an index of veridicality, which was simply the percentage of agreement between providers and receivers of support. Agreement was highest between each individual and those in his or her innermost circle, especially between husbands and wives. Agreement of people with those in their inner circle was 86 percent, and it ranged from 60 to 49 percent as one moved toward those in the outer circles.

Antonucci, T.C. (1986). Measuring social support networks: hierarchical mapping technique. *Generations* 10(4):10.

Cohen, S., et al. (1985). Measuring the functional components of social support. In Sarason, I.G., and Sarason, B., eds., *Social support: theory, research and application*, 73. The Hague, Holland: Martinus Niijhoff.

Kahn, R.L., and Antonucci, T.C. (1980). Convoys over the life course. In Baltes, P.B., and Brim, O.G., eds., *Life span development and behavior*, 253. New York: Academic Press.

Support in Old Age

Acitelli, L., and Antonucci, T.C. (1994). Gender differences in the link between marital support and satisfaction in older couples. *Journal of Personality and Social Psychology* 67(4):688.

Antonucci, T.C., and Israel, B. (1986). Veridicality of social support: a comparison of principal and network members' responses. *Journal of Consulting and Clinical Psychology* 54(4):432.

Antonucci, T.C., and Akiyama, H. (1987). An examination of sex differences in social support among older men and women. *Sex Roles* 17:737.

Antonucci, T.C., et al. (1990). Social support and reciprocity: a cross-ethnic and cross-national perspective. *Journal of Social and Personal Relationships* 7(4):519.

Ingersoll-Dayton, B., and Antonucci, T.C. (1988). Reciprocal and non-reciprocal social support: contrasting sides of intimate relationships. *Journal of Gerontology: Social Sciences* 43(3):S65.

Social Support and Health

Bosworth, H.B., and Schaie, K.W. (1997). The relationship of social environment, social networks, and health outcomes in the Seattle Longitudinal Study: two analytical approaches. *Journal of Gerontology:* Psychological Science 52B(5):197.

Garfein, A.J., and Herzog, A.R. (1995). Robust aging among the young-old, old-old, and oldest-old. *Journal of Gerontology: Social Sciences* 50B(2):S77.

Seeman, T.E., et al. (1994). Social ties and support and neuroendocrine function: the MacArthur studies of successful aging. *Annals of Behavioral Medicine* 16(2):95.

———. (1995). Behavioral and psychosocial predictors of physical performance: MacArthur studies of successful aging. *Journal of Gerontology: Medical Sciences* 50A(4):M177.

Uchino, B.N., et al. (1995). Appraisal support predicts age-related differences in cardiovascular function in women. *Health Psychology* 14(6):556.

———. (1995). *Beyond unidimensional conceptualizations of social support: specific dimensions of social support predict cellular immune function.* Unpublished manuscript.

Goodness of Fit

Avorn, J., and Langer, E.J. (1982). Induced disability in nursing home patients: a controlled trial. *Journal of the American Geriatric Society* 30(6):397.

Bandura, A. (1997). *Self-efficacy.* New York: Freeman.

The concept of self-efficacy, proposed by Albert Bandura, is similar to mastery, internal control, and several other terms that refer to an individual's belief that his or her efforts to perform certain tasks or achieve certain outcomes will be successful. Bandura's definition is task-specific and is central to his theory of cognition and motivation. The many experiments by him, his colleagues, and his students constitute an impressive demonstration of the importance of the concept and its relevance to the problems of everyday life—from overcoming phobias to enhancing mathematical performance.

This work is well summarized and a full bibliography is provided in Bandura's book, *Self-efficacy.*

Mendes de Leon, C.F., et al. (1996). Self-efficacy, physical decline, and change in functioning in community-living elders: a prospective study. *Journal of Gerontology: Social Sciences* 51B(4):S183.

Seeman, T.E., et al. (1996). Social network characteristics and onset of ADL disability: MacArthur studies of successful aging. *Journal of Gerontology: Social Sciences* 51B(4):S191.

Seligman, M.E. (1975). *Helplessness: on depression, development, and death.* San Francisco: Freeman.

The concept of learned helplessness was first proposed by Martin E.P. Seligman almost 30 years ago. Since that time, he and his colleagues have conducted many experiments demonstrating that animals (dogs and rats), if subjected to aversive stimuli (usually electric shock) under conditions that made escape or avoidance impossible, subsequently failed to escape even when escape became possible. Seligman concluded that they had learned to be helpless. The applicability of the concept to human beings was shown in experiments with college students as voluntary subjects [Hiroto, D.S., and Seligman, M.E. (1975). Generality of learned helplessness in man. *Journal of Personality and Social Psychology* 31(2):311].

CHAPTER II

Tennyson, A. (1937). Ulysses. In Lowry, H.F., and Thorp, W., eds., *Oxford anthology of English poetry.* New York: Oxford University Press.

The quotation is from lines 22–24 of that marvelous poem. Later lines are no less moving. The limitations of old age are acknowledged, but its continuing potential is asserted (lines 65–67):

Though much is taken, much abides; and though

We are not now that strength which in old days

Moved earth and heaven, that which we are, we are . . .

For citations and a discussion of the often quoted Freudian phrase on work and love, see:

Smelser, N.J. (1980). Issues in the study of work and love. In Smelser, N.J., and Erikson, E.H., eds., *Themes of work and love in adulthood,* 4. Cambridge, MA: Harvard University Press.

The Ambivalence of Society

The U.S. Bureau of the Census, both in the decennial census and in the monthly current population survey, defines work in terms of money income and excludes all unpaid work. The key question asks whether the respondent did any work for pay or profit during the preceding (or census) week. Anyone who answers "no" to this question is classified as a nonworker. The publications of the Census Bureau and the monthly data released by the U.S. Department of Labor are based on this definition. It is therefore built into the many derivative publications and policies that utilize census data.

This more comprehensive definition of productive activity, which emphasizes the creation of economic value rather than the receipt of pay, has now been used successfully in several large surveys in addition to the MacArthur community-based studies. It was first developed for Americans' Changing Lives, a nationwide study conducted by the Survey Research Center (University of Michigan) and supported by the National Institute on Aging.

It is also used in two other national surveys, the longitudinal Health and Retirement Study (HRS) and the related study of Asset and Health Dynamics Among the Oldest Old (AHEAD), both conducted by the Survey Research Center with the support of the National Institute on Aging.

For a more complete description of these studies, see:

Juster, F.T., and Suzman, R.M. (1995). An overview of the health and retirement study. *The Journal of Human Resources* 30(supplement):S7.

Myers, G.C. (guest editor). (1997). Asset and Health Dynamics Among the Oldest Old (AHEAD): initial results from the longitudinal study [special issue]. *Journals of Gerontology, Series B: Psychological and Social Sciences* 52B(May).

What Older People Really Do

André, R. (1981). *Homemakers, the forgotten workers.* Chicago: University of Chicago Press.

Garfein, A.J., and Herzog, A.R. (1995). Robust aging among the young-old, old-old, and oldest-old. *Journal of Gerontology: Social Sciences* 50B(2):S77.

Glass, T.A., et al. (1995). Change in productive activity in late adulthood: MacArthur studies of successful aging. *Journal of Gerontology: Social Sciences* 50B(2):S65.

Herzog, A.R., et al. (1989). Age differences in productive activities. *Journal of Gerontology: Social Sciences* 44(4):S129.

Herzog, A.R., and Morgan, J.N. (1992). Age and gender differences in the value of productive activities: four different approaches. *Research on Aging* 14:169.

Kahn, R.L. (1984). Productive behavior through the life course: an essay on the quality of life. *Human Resource Management* 23(1):5.

Morgan, J.N. (1986). Unpaid productive activity over the life course. In Institute of Medicine/National Research Council, eds., *Americans aging: productive roles in an older society.* Washington, DC: National Academy Press.

What It Takes To Be Productive

Findings on the predictors of continued productive activity in old age are based on the MacArthur studies in three areas: East Boston, New Haven, and Durham, North Carolina.

Bandura, A. (1997). *Self-efficacy: the exercise of control.* New York: Freeman.

———. (1997). Self-efficacy: toward a unifying theory of behavioral change. *Psychological Review* 84:191.

Albert Bandura, a cognitive psychologist at Stanford University, developed the concept of self-efficacy and has written extensively on the subject over many years. He defines self-efficacy as "people's beliefs in their capabilities to organize and execute the courses of action required to deal with prospective situations." As this definition suggests, Bandura considers self-efficacy a belief and that it is situation specific, or at least limited to specific domains of activity. The fact that I consider myself an excellent driver (high self-efficacy) does not imply that I also consider myself an excellent swimmer—or writer!

Other researchers have proposed related concepts, including internal control, mastery, and learned optimism. For a discussion of similarities and differences among them and for a summary of research findings, see:

Haidt, J., and Rodin, J. (1995). *Control and efficacy: an integrative review.* Report to the John D. and Catherine T. MacArthur Foundation Program on Mental Health and Human Development. Unpublished.

The Self-Fulfilling Prophecy and the Pygmalion Effect

The term "self-fulfilling prophecy" is almost self-explanatory, and the concept figures prominently in social/psychological research. It reminds us that, having made a prediction, we often act in ways that confirm it, that "make it come true." For further explication, see:

Merton, R. (1957). *Social theory and social structure.* New York: Free Press.

The underlying idea, however, goes back at least to Pascal, whose *Pensées* include the following lines: "Man is so made that by continually telling him he is a fool he believes it, and by continually telling it to himself he makes himself believe it. For man holds an inward talk with himself alone, in which it behooves him to regulate well."

Pascal, B. (1967). Quote # 536. In Stevenson, B., ed., *The home book of quotations: classical and modern*, 1788. New York: Dodd, Mead. (Reprinted from *Pensées*).

The most extensive line of research to test this broad proposition has concentrated on the "Pygmalion effect," which can be considered a special case of the self-fulfilling prophecy. Most of that research is experimental and has involved the behavior of teachers toward students, although some has involved leader behavior in other contexts. The dominant finding is that when teachers or other leaders are informed that particular individuals or groups are capable of unusually high performance, the leaders then act in ways that enable them to attain high performance. Key references include:

Eden, D. (1984). Self-fulfilling prophecy as a management tool: harnessing Pygmalion. *Academy of Management Review* 9(1):64.

Grieger, R. (1971). Pygmalion revisited: a loud call for caution. *Interchange* 2(4):78.

Rosenthal, R. (1973). The pygmalion effect lives. *Psychology Today* 7(4):56.

What Do Older People Want?

Most standard texts in survey research include discussions of social desirability bias and frame of reference. See, for example:

Kahn, R.L., and Cannell, C.F. (1957). *The dynamics of interviewing.* New York: Wiley.

Numerous "lie scales" have been devised to obtain estimates of the tendency of survey respondents to give "socially desirable" responses. Among the best known are the Marlowe-Crowne Social Desirability Scale and the Lie Scale of the Eyesenck Personality Questionnaire (EPQ). An extensive methodological literature has been generated around the use of such scales. Few of these studies include age as a variable, however. An exception is:

Ray, J.J. (1988). Lie scales and the elderly. *Personality and Individual Differences* 9(2):417.

In a series of Australian studies, 9 out of 11 showed significant positive correlations (.20 to .42) between age and scores on the Marlowe-Crowne Social Desirability Scale. These correlations were generated almost entirely by female respondents, however. Replications of this research in West Germany and India reported similar results.

"Oughts" and "Shoulds": The Question of Values

Responses to the "ought and should" questions are from Americans' Changing Lives. For a discussion of these value orientations, see:

Herzog, A.R., and House, J.S. (1991). Productive activities and aging well. *Generations* 15(Winter):49.

CHAPTER 12

Aesthetic and biographical writings on Whistler are numerous. A sample of them includes:

Anderson, R. (1995). *James McNeill Whistler: beyond the myth*. New York: Carroll and Graf.
Dorment, R. (1994). *James McNeill Whistler*. London: Tate Gallery.
Fleming, G.H. (1991). *James Abbott McNeill Whistler: a life*. New York: St. Martin's Press.
Prideaux, T. (1970). *The world of Whistler, 1834–1903*. New York: Time-Life Books.
Spalding, R. (1994). *Whistler*. London: Phaidon Press.
Taylor, H. (1978). *James McNeill Whistler*. New York: Putnam.
The Whistler papers. (1986). Lowell, MA: Whistler House Museum.

Changes in Life Expectancy

Olshansky, S.J. (1997). The demography of aging. In Cassel, C.K., et al., eds., *Geriatric Medicine*, 3rd ed. New York: Springer, 29–36.
Olshansky, S.J., and Ault, B. (1986). The fourth stage of the epidemiologic transition: the age of delayed degenerative diseases. *Milbank Quarterly* 64:355.
Rogers, R., and Hackenberg, R. (1989). Extending epidemiologic transition theory: a new stage. *Social Biology* 34(3–4):234.

Some Implications of Longer Life

Bortz, W.M. (1991). *We live too short and die too long*. New York: Bantam.
Katz, S., et al. (1983). Active life expectancy. *New England Journal of Medicine* 309:1218.
Olshansky, S.J., et al. (1990). In search of Methuselah: stimulating the upper limits of human longevity. *Science*, 250:634.

Soldo, B.J., et al. (May 1997). Asset and health dynamics among the oldest old: an overview of the AHEAD baseline (special issue). In Myers, G.C. (Guest ed.), *Journal of Gerontology, Series B: Psychological and Social Sciences* 52B (1).

Taeuber, C.M. (1992). Sixty-five plus in America. *Current population reports P23–178RV.* U.S. Bureau of the Census.

Older Men and Women: Asset or Burden?

Barth, M.C., et al. (1995). Older Americans as workers. In Bass, S.A., ed., *Older and active: how Americans over 55 are contributing to society,* 35. New Haven, CT: Yale University Press.

Lubitz, J., et al. (1995). Longevity and Medicare expenditures. *New England Journal of Medicine* 332(15):999.

Riley, G.F., and Lubitz, J.D. (1993). Trends in Medicare payments in the last year of life. *New England Journal of Medicine* 328:1092.

Rowe, J.W. (1996). Health care myths at the end of life. *Bulletin of the American College of Surgeons* 81(6):11.

Actual and Potential: Prospects for Increased Productivity

Caro, F.G., and Bass, S.A. (1995). Increasing volunteering among older people. In Bass, S.A., ed., *Older and active: how Americans over 55 are contributing to society,* 71. New Haven, CT: Yale University Press.

Garfein, A.J., and Herzog, A.R. (1995). Robust aging among the young-old, old-old, and oldest-old. *Journal of Gerontology: Social Sciences* 50B(2):S77.

Harris, L., and Associates. (1992). *Aging in the eighties: America in transition.* Washington, DC: National Council on the Aging.

Herzog, A.R., et al. (1989). Age differences in productive activities. *Journal of Gerontology: Social Sciences* 44(4):S129.

Realizing the Potential: What Will It Take?

Baltes, P.B. (1997). On the incomplete architecture of human ontogeny. *American Psychologist* 52(4):366.

Burgess, E. (1957). The older generation and the family. In Donahue, W., and Tibbits, C., eds., *The new frontiers of aging,* 158. Ann Arbor, MI: University of Michigan Press.

The Einstein quotation was cited in *Beyond War,* a bulletin of the Foundation for Global Community in Palo Alto, CA. Einstein's views on nuclear weapons are reiterated in many of his writings, including:

Einstein, A. *Einstein on peace.* (1963). London: Methuen.
———. *Out of my later years.* (1967). Totowa, NJ: Littlefield Adams.

————. *The collected papers of Albert Einstein.* (1987–). Princeton, NJ: Princeton University Press.

————. *The quotable Einstein.* (1996). Princeton, NJ: Princeton University Press.

Kahn, R.L. (1984). Productive behavior through the life course: an essay on the quality of life. *Human Resource Management* 23(1):5.

Riley, M.W., and Riley, J.W. (1994). Structural lag: past and future. In Riley, M.W., et al., eds., *Age and structural lag: society's failure to provide meaningful opportunities in work, family, and leisure,* 15. New York: John Wiley.

In 1881 the German chancellor Otto von Bismarck proposed a program of national retirement pensions, health insurance, and accident insurance. All were approved by the Reichstag. Shortly after the turn of the century, David Lloyd George led a successful campaign for a similar program in Great Britain. A generation later, the New Deal administration of Franklin D. Roosevelt enacted the Social Security program of the United States. For perspective on these developments, see:

Rose, J. (1985). From Bismarck to Roosevelt: how the welfare state began (teachers' ed.). *Scholastic Update* 118:13.

United States Committee on Economic Security. (1937). *Social Security in America: the factual background of the Social Security Act as summarized from staff reports to the Committee on Economic Security.* Washington, DC: U.S. Government Printing Office.

Concepts of the Life Course

Neugarten, B.L. (1974). Age groups in American society and the rise of the young-old. *Annals of the American Academy of Political and Social Science* 320:187.

Pifer, A., and Bronte, L., eds. (1986). *Our aging society: paradox and promise.* New York: Norton.

Methods of Social Accounting

For a more extended discussion of the place of statistical data in policy formation, see:

Campbell, A. (1981). *The sense of well-being in America: recent patterns and trends.* New York: McGraw-Hill.

Education, Work, and Leisure

Riley M., and Riley, J. (1994). Structural lag: past and future. In Riley, M., et al., eds., *Age and structural lag.* New York: Wiley-Interscience.

Schorr, J.B. (1991). *The overworked American.* New York: Basic Books.

Policies for the Future: Getting from Here to There

Bass, S.A., et al. (1995). Toward pro-work policies and programs for older Americans. In Bass, S.A., ed., *Older and active: how Americans over 55 are contributing to society,* 263. New Haven, CT: Yale University Press.

Butler, R.N. (1997). Living longer, contributing longer. *Journal of the American Medical Association* 278(16):1372.

Campbell, D.T. (1969). Reforms as experiments. *American Psychologist* 24(4):409.

Older Americans Act, Title IV & Title V.

Quinn, R.P., and Staines, G.L. (1979). *The 1977 quality of employment survey.* Ann Arbor, MI: Institute for Social Research.

The Work Module

Planned organizational change is, of course, a subject of continuing interest to top corporate managers, other organizational leaders, and the many consultants who advise them. It is also a subject that has generated a large literature, some of it research-based, much of it of the "how-to" variety. Research-based examples include:

Dunnette, M.D. and Hough, L.M., eds. (1992). *Handbook of industrial and organizational psychology.* Palo Alto, CA: Consulting Psychologists Press. See volume 3, sections 2 and 3, especially Porras, J.I., and Robertson, P.J., Organizational development: theory, practice, and research, p. 719.

Katz, D. and Kahn, R.L. (1978). *The social psychology of organizations.* New York: Wiley. See chapter 19, Organizational change; chapter 20, Convergences and combinations. Scott, W.R. (1992). *Organizations: rational, natural, and open systems.* Englewood Cliffs, NJ: Prentice Hall. See chapter 9, Boundary setting and boundary spanning.

The concept of the work module originated in conversations with Leslie Kish. For a fuller exposition of this topic, see Kahn, R.L. (1974). The work module: a proposal for the humanization of work. In J. O'Toole, ed., *Work and the quality of life: resource papers for work in America.* Cambridge, MA: MIT Press.

INDEX

ABOUT THE AUTHORS

John W. Rowe, M.D., is president of the Mount Sinai School of Medicine and Mount Sinai Hospital in New York City. Dr. Rowe has chaired the MacArthur Foundation Research Network on Successful Aging since its inception and is a member of the Institute of Medicine of the National Academy of Sciences. He is fifty-three and lives in New York City.

Robert L. Kahn, Ph.D., is professor emeritus of psychology and public health at the University of Michigan, where he is also research scientist emeritus at the Institute for Social Research. He is a member of the MacArthur Foundation Research Network on Successful Aging and a member of the American Academy of Arts and Sciences. He is eighty and lives in Ann Arbor, Michigan.